Penelope Williams grew up in Carleton Place and Ottawa, studied at the University of Toronto and worked at the University of Toronto Press. In 1983 she started her own writing and editing business, PMF Editorial Services Inc., in Ottawa. After a breast cancer diagnosis in 1988, she wrote about her experiences in *That Other Place: A Personal Account of Breast Cancer*, which went on to win the Ottawa Carleton Book Award. She is a member of the Founders Circle of Willow Breast Cancer Support Canada and was on the advisory committee for the Ontario Breast Cancer Community Research Initiative. She and her husband live in Westport, Ontario.

BREAST CANCER

BIOGRAPHY OF AN ILLNESS

PENELOPE WILLIAMS

Published in 2008 by
BPS books
Toronto, Canada
www.bpsbooks.net
A division of Bastian Publishing Services Ltd.

First published as Breast Cancer: Landscape of an Illness in 2004 by Penguin Group (Canada)

Author representation: Westwood Creative Artists
94 Harbord St., Toronto, Ontario M5S 1G6

Library and Archives Canada Cataloguing in Publication

Williams, Penelope M., 1943–
Breast cancer: biography of an illness/Penelope Williams

ISBN 978-0-9809231-5-5

1. Breast—Cancer—Popular works. I. Title.

RC280.B8W49 2008   616.99'449   C2008-904102-X

Cover design: Greg Devitt Design

For Nicole Bruinsma

CONTENTS

ACKNOWLEDGMENTS

THIS IS A BOOK that at first I had not wanted to write—another book about breast cancer, a tough and searing subject. I didn't want to go there again, in any sense. But people and events changed all that pretty quickly, and it has been an extraordinary experience.

Nicole Bruinsma was the inspiration to wade once again into the lists of this disease. You will meet her here and see why. You will see her courage and indomitable determination, her grace and compassion, her wit and huge heart. All the time I have been working on this book, it's as if I've been in her company. It has been a privilege and often been hard, and I am so very grateful to Scott Findlay, her husband and my nephew, for making it possible. I thank him for sharing his memories and his insights, for his jokes, for his gentle course corrections and for his endless patience in explaining the science. If there are mistakes here, they are mine in interpretation, not his in explanation.

I thank all the women who took the time and energy, often in short supply, to tell their stories. As well as reading their words in these pages, I hope you can hear their voices, hear the courage and humour, the pain, poignancy, irony, anger and the honesty there. Their generosity is a gift that might lift a little the loneliness of others who find themselves on the same journey. Most of these women wanted their own names used. The few pseudonyms are identified by the use of an initial instead of a last name.

An apology is due here to all men who have or have had breast cancer. You are in the minority, but that doesn't lessen the impact of the disease; in fact, maybe it just intensifies it by the isolation you must feel in an environment focused so exclusively on women's experiences. In these pages please understand that in most instances "she" and "her" can mean "he" and "his" as well.

I thank the physicians who carved time out of very busy schedules to talk about their experiences on the breast cancer wards; they spoke about their frustrations, about their dreams that someday they will be able to ensure with certainty that every woman and every man with the disease can get better. They provide a view of breast cancer from the other side; their perceptions bring a balance to understanding the huge challenges in fighting this disease on all levels.

For their exuberant support and trenchant advice in the earliest days of this book, I thank my friends Sue Wright, Falia Damianakis, Judy Gould, Chris Sinding and Carol Burnham Cook. At a brainstorming session at the Third World Conference on Breast Cancer in Victoria, B.C., in June 2002, a meeting full of passion, intelligence and laughter, they gave me direction and a wish list of what this book should encompass. One said that it should be a kind of navigational aid and that "as we go along, it should incorporate . . . please note, Penny, now it's *we,* now it's *our* book." I hope that after seeing the finished version they still want it to be their book.

My deep appreciation to the OBC-CRI and the members of its advisory committee. Behind this daunting acronym (it stands for the Ontario Breast Cancer Community Research Initiative) is an extraordinary group of young researchers led by Ross Gray and Margaret Fitch. Their work on the psychosocial issues facing women with breast cancer is so rich and relevant and accessible, I wanted to include all of it. What I learned from them informs much of the discussion here.

My thanks to Elodie d'Ombrain for arranging interviews with patients, social workers and physicians in Moncton, New Brunswick, undaunted by the fact that the entire city appeared to be away on holiday the week I was there; Dianne Perrier for, once again, keeping PMF Editorial Services going and for coming up with information reported in places I would never have thought of looking; Hilary McMahon for being the most supportive and encouraging agent and friend; Andrea Crozier for wanting someone to write not just about breast cancer, the disease, but about all the issues and controversies it comes wrapped in and believing that I could be that someone; and Don Bastian of BPS Books for believing that this book "has legs" and should continue to be out there to help and inform anyone touched by breast cancer.

Finally, and again, huge thanks and gratitude to all my family, especially my sons, Matt and Sam and their Erin(n)s, for their endless encouragement and support, and my husband, Allen Sackmann, who got to hear every wandering thought and theory, who listened patiently to my rants and doubts, who had the wisdom to know when to offer advice and the self-preservation to know when to keep very quiet indeed. He has been my sounding board, punching bag and chief supporter.

INTRODUCTION

B<small>REAST CANCER IS A DEADLY DISEASE</small>, even if you don't die of it. It was 50 years ago, it was in 2004 when this book was originally published under the title, *Breast Cancer: Landscape of an Illness*, and it still is in 2008. Despite the improving survival rates, it still kills. Much of its menace, and the reason that a diagnosis strikes with the numbing force of a death sentence, is its unpredictability. It kills— or doesn't—with impunity, choosing its victims with the malevolence of a capricious sniper. The very randomness of a breast cancer "hit" strikes fear in all its possible victims. We can crouch behind healthy living, take shelter in a family tree free of the breast cancer genes or hide within a mantle of youth, but the breast cancer bullet can still find us. Like frustrated cops trying to fathom the pattern of the sniper's behaviour and foil his next move, researchers look for the clues, the patterns, the genes, the markers that will tell them who will get the disease, who will be felled by it, who will survive it, and how that knowledge can be used to prevent or cure the disease altogether.

This has not happened yet. Despite the steady outpouring of magazine articles and newspaper headlines touting breakthroughs in treatment, the upbeat cancer drug advertisements that feature terrifyingly healthy women, the promises that prevention and early detection will keep you cancer free and the annual salvos of the more optimistic fundraisers that "breast cancer can be beaten," it can't be, not for everyone, not all the time. The coupling of prevention with early detection is particularly puzzling, a kind of oxymoron that flows through the literature virtually unchallenged. The sad reality is, no matter how early a cancer is detected, it has not been prevented. Once you've detected it, you've got it, too late to prevent it.

Over the last several years, public attention to breast cancer has been brought to humming pitch mainly by the growing involvement of cancer patients themselves. And, as one friend comments, "The hum is not always harmonious." The world of breast cancer is fraught with issues, and until real cures are found, the debates around these issues will continue to swirl.

A breast cancer diagnosis hurls you out of the old and familiar and into the new and scary, and very likely without warning. As is the case for so many women, your body might not have given you any inkling that something was amiss. You felt just fine, no pain or fatigue presaged the diagnosis, so you went cold turkey into the world of the sick without even *feeling* sick. Now, you find yourself adjusting priorities, reassessing everything you took for granted before, learning new skills to get through each day — in fact, rewriting yourself to fit into this harsh new context. Your life is governed by a whole new set of imperatives and you find you have no training to deal with them and no academic distancing to buffer yourself against the insidious myths, the cold facts and the soupy confusion into which you have been so suddenly thrust. The reality is that these are now part of your world, not someone else's.

The burden of the physical disease is hard enough — the treatments that invade your body one way or another, the short leash of weekly or even daily hospital appointments, the anxiety of waiting for test results. It is made worse when you discover the controversies that shroud this disease. These are the debates about risk factors, early detection and diagnostic techniques, about alternative therapies, doctor-patient relationships and patients' responsibilities; the criticisms of the clinical trial process; the questioning of the motives and honesty of pharmaceutical companies; and the frustration of dealing with conflicting study results on the efficacy and safety of a new drug or treatment approach, a drug that you might be on, or a treatment you might have just completed;

and the scandals that erupt way too often about mistakes and cover-ups in the labs and medical wards, and now even in the corridors of politics. It can be overwhelming.

If your cancer spreads from the breast to the bones, the liver, the lungs, the brain, it is still called breast cancer but with the chilling qualifiers "advanced" or "metastatic." The breast is its primary site, but now the cancer cells are attacking organs vital to life. Now you must deal with the same issues but at a far starker and more immediate intensity.

In the introduction to the 2004 edition of this book I wrote that it became sadly clear that keeping up with breaking developments was not the challenge I thought it would be, that although some of the details might change, the big issues had a depressing constancy about them.

They are all part of the line dance of breast cancer, I wrote, "where some weeks the pattern is one step forward, two steps back, and other weeks, it's two steps forward, one step back, though the dancers stay more or less in the same place."

It is five years later, and although the dancers may feel like they are marking time, shuffling on the same worn spot, in fact there is movement forward. Granted, there have been few eureka moments — we're still a long way from nailing the cause(s) and the cure(s) — but it's not through lack of trying. Researchers are looking everywhere — at genes and their mutations, at viruses and vaccines, at new diagnostic methods, improved radiation therapies, new surgical procedures, new chemos, new ways of delivering therapeutics, new generations of hormonal treatments, new combination therapies, and targetted therapies customized to an individual patient's needs. If progress can be measured in energy and commitment, and in small incremental steps, then there has assuredly been progress. On some issues. On others it's still round and round the houses — circular and seemingly endless angry debates that pull into their vortex of conflicting information the very people who need clarity the most.

Risk factors continue to be confused with cause; some we cannot avoid, some are used as big sticks to encourage us to alter our lifestyles, some are myths that shouldn't be on the list in the first place. Abortion is still out there as a "cause," a heartbreaking piece of misinformation that can bring a woman so much additional pain wrapped in guilt. Some risk factors go on and off the list like yo-yos. Alcohol, for example, is back on. A National Cancer Institute (US) study, the results of which were released in 2008, found that specific variations within two genes involved with alcohol metabolism are associated with an increased risk of breast cancer in post-menopausal women who drank as little as "one small glass" a day in earlier years. "The higher their alcohol consumption, the higher their risk," says the lead author of the study. But wait. Before you start to despair about your dissolute early years, she goes on to say that the work needs to be explored further and replicated by other studies. This is the way of science; a slow and careful progression of repeats to support a hypothesis. It is easy to grab at such an announcement, very much in its early days, and drastically alter your lifestyle, or beat yourself up over an old one, only to read two months later another announcement to the effect, "Wrong. A new study finds no connection between moderate alcohol intake and risk of developing breast cancer." You can end up feeling like a ball in a particularly aggressive ping pong match. It is really hard to identify the signposts in the risk factor sea of information that actually stand firm for more than a few months. The neon one is incontrovertible: simply being a woman.

It is difficult to fathom that Breast Self-Examination (BSE), such a commonsense approach to detecting changes in your breasts, could be controversial. It is and continues to be. In 2006, the Breast Disease Committee of the Society of Obstetricians and Gynaecologists of Canada recommended that women should not be taught BSE, flying straight in the face of the instinctive belief of most women that they know their own bodies best and would be the first to recognize any changes. In 2008, the National Cancer Institute (US) reinforced the findings of earlier studies that BSE does not reduce women's risk of dying from breast cancer and in fact it could be harmful because of the stress caused by finding non-existent or benign lumps.

The discussion continues over the efficacy of screening mammography, but proponents offer the telling argument that survival rates in Canada started to improve shortly after screening mammography programs were introduced in this country, suggesting that early detection is working. The debate that continues loudest is about screening mammograms for women between the ages of 40 and 49. The National Cancer Institute (US), the American Cancer Society and the American College of Radiology now recommend annual screening mammograms for women in that age group despite the opinion of many researchers and doctors who say it is not a good idea. In 2007, Dr. Cornelia Baines from University of Toronto and Dr Steven Groopman from the School of Public Health, Johns Hopkins University, among others, both said screening mammograms for women in their 40s do more harm than good because of false negatives and because they can pick up pseudo disease (small tumours that may or may not become cancer) leading to unnecessary lumpectomies or mastectomies; they add that mammograms are not as effective for younger women anyway because of their denser breast tissue and can be harmful in exposing menstruating women to radiation.

The Canadian Cancer Society and Canadian Breast Cancer Network continue to recommend screening mammography for women between the ages of 50 and 69 although some studies published in 2008 indicate that it is also beneficial for women over 70. Earlier detection in this age group — finding tumours at a "non-invasive stage" — would minimize surgical procedures and improve prognosis.

Controversy still lingers around the use of hormonal therapies as prevention for women at high risk of developing breast cancer but who are healthy in all respects. They are not benign drugs and do have side effects. Their use in prevention of recurrence is standard treatment now, but it can be a challenge to find current and unbiased data about the various therapies on offer in this area. Indeed, the internet has become even more of a jungle of conflicting and misinformation than five years ago. Let's say, for instance, that you have had surgery, chemo and radiation treatment for primary cancer, and now your doctor recommends that you take a hormone therapy for the next five years. You have been told that you are in danger of developing osteoporosis and someone tells you about Raloxifene (marketed as Evista), a drug used for the treatment of osteoporosis that also seemed to show promise in the treatment of breast cancer. Sounds like a good choice for you. You do an internet search and this is what you find.

In June 2006, an early release article on the initial results of the STAR trial (comparing Raloxifene with Tamoxifen) stated that Raloxifene was "preferable" to Tamoxifen for breast cancer prevention. In October of that same year, researchers at Duke University sounded a note of caution about Raloxifene in a letter to the *New England Journal of Medicine*. Despite such reservations, in 2007, the US Food and Drug Administration (FDA) approved it for use in breast cancer prevention. But when you check the Canadian Clinical Practice Guidelines for the Care and Treatment of Breast Cancer (Questions and Answers for Women), you read: "One drug used to treat osteoporosis that is not recommended for women who have had breast cancer is raloxifene, a selective estrogen receptor modulator." This guideline was last updated in April 2002, so you think, 'OK, it just hasn't been updated yet.' But, and here is the catch, we are told that these guidelines are reviewed and updated every six months by a steering committee because they are used by doctors for guidance in recommending therapies for their patients. So is raloxifene in or out? Who knows. Wikipedia says this: "There has been criticism in the mainstream oncology press of the way that [the FDA approval] information about the drug was released. There has been some confusion in the lay media about the meaning of the trial results. There is no specific clinical evidence for the use of raloxifene in the adjuvant treatment of breast cancer over established drugs such as tamoxifen or anastrozole."

Scandals in the breast cancer world are not commonplace but they still continue to surface with an astonishing similarity in their trajectories from rumour, through denial, cover-up and finally exposure. Whether the elements of the scandal originate in botched tests in a lab, fraudulent practices of an individual doctor or unethical activities at a corporate level, they all have a crushing impact on one of the most important elements of the relationship between a patient and the medical community: trust.

In July 2007 a Commission of Inquiry on Hormone Receptor Testing was established by the Government of Newfoundland and Labrador to find out why more than 1,000 breast cancer patients who underwent hormone receptor testing between 1997 and 2005 in that province had to be retested, why it took so long to contact the women involved, and why awareness of the problem took seven years to surface. Of the 1,013 patients retested, more than a third had been given the wrong results. Because they were deemed to be estrogen/progesterone-negative but actually weren't, 383 patients were denied anti-hormonal therapies clinically shown to improve a patient's odds of survival. More than 100 of these patients are now dead. The inquiry discovered that two years after the faulty lab work came to light, 44 patients had still not been contacted despite the bureaucracy's emphatic claims to the contrary.

In the midst of all this, the blame game kicked in. Politicians waffled about when they had been told about the problem, accusing managers at the Eastern Health Authority for giving bad advice and for obfuscation. The CEO of the Authority resigned over the affair after it became obvious that his staff and senior managers didn't seem to get it, blaming bad publicity for the growing scandal rather than bad lab work and their own worse follow-up. In 2005, when the problem first surfaced, a spokesperson allegedly wanted to "hold off" a reporter's queries, writing in an internal memo: "That way, the issue should be dead again by the time the House opens again next week." Sadly, so would many breast cancer patients who had missed out on the proper treatment because of the botched tests. In such circumstances, trust really takes a hit, as do the breast cancer patients who fall victim not just to the disease but to the very system that they believe will help them fight it.

On a more positive note, there is real if slow progress in therapeutic research. "Slow" of course is relative: to a woman hoping for new treatments to stem her cancer, all advances seem painfully, diabolically sluggish. To researchers looking everywhere and at everything that could possibly prevent, retard or cure the disease, the pace must be deliberate and painstaking. It is a prerequisite of the scientific method, and some say it is beginning to pay off and that there is cause for cautious optimism.

Historically, breast cancer treatments have been "one-size-fits-all," but the problem is they *don't* fit all, because breast cancer is not a single disease. The growing recognition of its heterogeneity, and the need to isolate predictive factors that would allow for customizing therapy are changing the approach to treatments. The challenges here are how to match the therapy to the individual patient, and the enormous cost of doing so. Dr. Pamela Goodwin, clinician-scientist at Mount Sinai Hospital, Toronto said in 2001 that in 10 years such targetted therapies might be the standard where the precise characteristics of a tumour would dictate the kind of treatment an individual receives. Seven years later and we are not there yet, but targetted approaches and customized treatments are certainly the wave of the nearer future.

Recent advances in microarray technology could revolutionize clinical practice; scientists can now study genes to identify "genetic signatures" of individuals which then could be matched with a specific therapy. In 2008, researchers at McGill University, Montreal, announced that they have drawn up one of the most detailed genetic profiles of breast cancer yet compiled, focusing on 26 genes that could be used to predict how patients would respond to different treatments. However, this approach is not without its wrinkles (see discussion of Herceptin below).

Biological therapies use the body's own immune system in one way or another to act on cancer cells while leaving healthy cells untouched. Researchers are actively studying the two arms of the immune response:

humoral (antibody production) and cellular (production of macrophages, natural killer cells, etc.). Monoclonals such as Herceptin (trastuzumab) use antibodies to attack cancer cells, and other immuno-therapies, for example dendritic cell therapies, target the cellular arm. Herceptin already has an established role in treatment, either as a single agent or in combination with chemotherapies. It seems to act in three ways: it sticks to special receptors on cancer cells to stop them from growing; it signals the body's own natural killer cells to attack cancer cells; and it works with chemotherapies to prevent cancer cells damaged by chemo from repairing themselves. Until recently, it was thought that Herceptin worked only in patients with the Her2Neu gene (about 15 to 20 percent of breast cancers have an amplification of this gene or overexpression of its protein, both leading to a worse prognosis), but it now appears to be effective as well in patients who do not overexpress the Her2Neu protein. This is good news for all breast cancer patients. In the meantime, researchers are looking for other mechanisms that must be at play here.

Viruses are another area of intense study. A Canadian scientist from Ottawa, Dr. John Bell, has been working on an oncolytic virus that is showing great promise. An oncolytic virus kills tumour cells by lysing (bursting apart) the cell membrane while leaving normal cells unharmed. The challenge, among many, is to fool the body's immune system into letting the virus past its defences to get at the cancer cells. Although China approved an oncolytic virus for the treatment of head and neck cancer in 2006, viruses are not in clinical practice here yet, although Dr. Bell's virus, as well as a number of others, is in clinical trials. He is optimistic about the future of this area of research: "What the whole field of oncolytic viruses needs is one good clinical trial that shows that this concept will work convincingly, and I think we're getting close now," Bell says. "Once that happens I think it will blow the doors off the field and everybody will jump in."

"Targetting" in a slightly different sense is a feature of advances in both chemotherapy and radiation, specifically in their delivery. In the field of chemotherapy, a plethora of new drugs and the way they are administered are in clinical trials now. However, when you read the clinical trial results as published for the lay public, it is often difficult to separate real progress from a chimera. The Internet is sprinkled with announcements of huge and exciting breakthroughs but when you read carefully you find that often these "eureka" discoveries are either puff pieces by pharmaceutical companies for their own drugs, or popular press headlines with no follow-up. The more reliable websites do include genuine developments over the last 10 or 12 years but always with the qualifier that more research is needed. One promising new taxane chemotherapy, Abraxane™, was approved for metastatic breast cancer treatment in Canada in 2007. Because it is delivered right to the tumour cells, higher doses can be administered without the need for toxic solvents, which are often the cause of the severe side effects of other taxane chemos.

There have also been advances in targetted radiation therapy. Intensity Modulated Radiation Therapy (IMRT) is a new technique that aims more radiation to the tumour site than to the surrounding tissue, thus reducing collateral damage. Computer-generated images calculate the dosage to each part of the breast, blocking the radiation beam during delivery to prevent "hot spots" in healthy tissue. The number of sessions and dosages assigned to each patient depends on the type, location and size of the tumour as well as the patient's age and overall health. A friend who has recently had this treatment described how when she looked into the eye of the machine, she was sure she could see the outline of the cavity left by her surgery, and rods sliding back and forth to direct the radiation. "They line me up with some beams (kind of like the laser beam on a table saw) and then zap me from each side," she wrote, then added wistfully, "I'll ask about it tomorrow but it would be [more] interesting if it wasn't being done on *my* boob." She had 16 sessions instead of the standard 25, and although she still suffered fatigue and skin burn she recovered more quickly than she might have done with the conventional treatment.

This book is for all those women who have joined the breast cancer club ... who must decide how active they are going to be on their journey, and who want to know about the implications of the discussions out there to make personal decisions.

But more than that, this book is for everyone who has been touched by the malevolent mystery of breast cancer, directly or indirectly, because the mysteries and pain of this disease are at some level mysteries and pain for all of us: women worried about getting it, women who have had it once and worry about getting it again, women who get it again and know that now they will not be free of it, men who get it, doctors who treat it, researchers who study it, fundraisers, volunteers, and activists who work and fight the disease in the public arena and policy-makers who direct government responses and responsibilities.

I write from the point of view of an involved participant and a first-hand observer. I am a 20-year breast cancer veteran informed by a personal battle with the disease, as well as through direct experience with much of its baggage, the hidden trappings I never knew existed until I found myself tangled in them. These are what so often bring an extra level of pain, anger and confusion to those already buckling under the weight of their physical disease.

The book is loosely constructed as the stages of a journey from pre- to post diagnosis, through treatment for primary and advanced disease, into the other territory that comes with breast cancer. And it tells the stories of women on this journey.

One of the biggest comforts in this new territory is the powerful camaraderie and shared experiences among women who have had or have the disease, especially those experiences that seem to go unacknowledged in the medical, public and political corridors of breast cancer. These form the strongest fabric of community. It's what we talk about at lunch or over a drink at the conferences rather than what is covered at the official sessions that reveal the true face of breast cancer. It's the joy of inclusion, when you find out you are not the only one whose breast cancer journey hasn't unfolded the way so many books or pamphlets say it will or should. The biography of breast cancer is in their stories, in their courage, their humour, their generosity, their pain, their dying and their living. They are why I wrote this book, stitched through with women's experiences that are, stripped to the basics, the real story, the only story, of breast cancer.

Penelope Williams
July 2008

1 | THE BLACK CATS OF BREAST CANCER: RISK FACTORS AND MYTHS

*Looking for the cause of cancer is like looking
in a dark room for a black cat that isn't there.*
—Geoff Conklin, *Scientific American*[1]

N<small>ICOLE PHONED VERY EARLY</small> one morning from her hospital bed. It was still dark, a February darkness that held no promise of spring, or even of light.

"I've joined your club, Pen," she said.

The club, of course, was breast cancer, a club that is becoming less and less exclusive. It will accept anyone as a member, and not one, not a single one, ever wanted to join.

It is a very old club: breast cancer has been around forever—evidence of it has turned up in Egyptian papyri dating back to 2500 B.C. But it's been a secret club up to the last two or three decades. Until about 15 years ago, breast cancer as the cause of death was seldom made public; obituaries rarely defined the cancer that killed more women than any other cancer.

"I had a mastectomy last night," Nicole said. "Could you come over?"

1

I got breast cancer, or it got me, in September 1988. The results of a second needle biopsy, contradicting the first one three months earlier that had given me the all clear, came in the middle of a week of family festivities in preparation for Nicole Bruinsma's marriage to my nephew Scott Findlay. I had stage 2 breast cancer, with two lymph nodes infected. The size of the tumour and number of lymph nodes involved was at that time considered stage 3 in the US. This was my first intimation that information in this new world was not fixed, certain and confirmable.

During my months of treatment and tests and appointments in which the doctors disagreed with each other over what I needed next, I would consult my own medical saviour, Nicole, who was a GP. I'd reel home from the cancer clinic brimming with data I didn't understand and, consequently, in the space of two kilometres and half an hour, manage to transform the perhaps originally clear information into gibberish. And I'd phone Nicole and whisper, "Help."

And she did, every time. Her honest explanations gave me the clarity I needed to feel less out of control—at least until the next appointment. She filtered out the grit of misunderstanding, mishearing and misinformation and crushed the boulders of fear into pebbles. She did this for me over and over again, until the boulders and grit stopped burying me like backfill on a construction site. She was my own personal navigator.

Now, nine years later, Nicole was embarking on the same journey, with the same stage of breast cancer, same sized tumour, same number of lymph nodes involved. At least that was according to the original report from the pathologist. On a closer look, it was established that three nodes had cancer cells in them. Now it was my turn; I could help, not by providing information—she already had that, and she knew well how to navigate the system—but by offering the one important thing I had. Through my own survival so far, I could give her hope.

Nicole was 37, with three young daughters, the year of her diagnosis. She worked in the local hospital, while maintaining her private practice at a clinic nearby. She worked hard, she played hard—Nicole was a serious athlete, hiking, swimming, paddling, skiing—she lived life to the fullest. And she was now about to live even harder and fuller.

Nicole had had a couple of scares, the most recent the summer before, but both times the lumps proved to be cysts. In the fall of 1996, she found another lump. Given her history it was easy to assume that this one would be a cyst too. She monitored the lump for a few weeks. It started to hurt (yet another case refuting the myth still loose in many GPs' examining rooms that if a lump hurts, it's not cancer). In early January 1997, she had a biopsy, and then scarpered to a yoga camp in the Bahamas with her daughters. The results were waiting for her when she returned at the end of the month. The lump was not a cyst; it was cancer. She acted quickly and within days had surgery.

Before the operation, she told Scott, "If [the surgeon] gets in there and finds bad news, tell her to go ahead with a mastectomy. Tell her to get it all, right now."

The surgeon went "in there," and while Nicole was still under anaesthetic on the operating table, sent tissue to the pathology lab. She came to Scott in the waiting room: "It's multifocal disease, Scott. It's throughout the breast." A lumpectomy was no longer an option. Scott gave the go-ahead for a full mastectomy with lymph node excision to assess if the disease had spread from the breast. Even though Nicole had told him that was what she wanted, emotionally, it was a searing decision to have to make for his wife. Medically, it was the only choice.

Surgery, February 27; home, February 28; a six-kilometre walk, March 2. This is Nicole we're talking about, after all. This was how she dealt with adversity—head on, head up. With Scott and her three daughters—Anneke, age seven; Aiden, age four; and Saraya, age two—she hiked up Penguin Hill to a log cabin in Gatineau Park, a refuge, a still point, in the widening gyre for many of our family. Then she walked home and chipped ice off the garage floor.

Later that week, she and Scott went to the Ottawa Regional Cancer Centre to see an oncologist. She wrote at the time, "I had felt quite cocky up until then but entering those hallowed halls drove home the reality of *me* being the patient."

The next day she went back to see the surgeon who was filling in for her own doctor, away on holiday. He didn't yet have the pathology report on how many lymph nodes were cancerous but didn't think this was all that crucial. "You already know you have node-positive disease," he said. "What more do you want to know?" Nicole was furious: "How *many* nodes, that's what I want to know, you idiot."

She also didn't know whether enough nodes had been taken out during her surgery—four were insufficient for a proper assessment of disease spread. The doctor mumbled something about if the surgeon only got four nodes, then that meant there *were* only four nodes. Nicole's comment was fairly succinct: Bullshit. She tracked down the pathologist who had first given her the bad news about at least one node being positive—"A nervous fellow," recalled Nicole, "he nearly jumped out of his skin when he saw me but told me that he now had found only two nodes positive." Out of how many, she asked him, still fearing the worst. The number of nodes affected mattered, really mattered, because the more nodes with cancer in them, the greater the likelihood the cancer had spread to other parts of the body. Doctors know this, lots of patients don't—at first. Nicole did. She recounted the conversation: "He said, 'I can't remember—let's count,' walks over to my slides and nonchalantly counts . . . nine. Whew. He then became quite chatty. I don't believe I heard or understood much of what was said after that—I was flying high—I was invincible, only two nodes!"

From a standing start, Nicole went into full throttle. With their scientific background, hers in medicine, his in biology, Nicole and Scott combined forces and tackled her illness with the ferocity and focus of a pair of tigers on a hunt. They interviewed oncologists, studied clinical trial results, enlisted colleagues in their research to ensure that she had the best treatment available.

That year, Nicole and I went together to the First World Conference on Breast Cancer, held in Kingston, Ontario, at Queen's

University, Nicole's alma mater. Just as it had been the first time she went to the Ottawa Regional Cancer Centre as a patient, it was deeply disturbing for her to be in this unexpected role, no longer a student looking forward to life but a cancer patient trying to hang onto it.

Nicole was in the middle of her chemotherapy treatments that June, and most of her lovely blonde hair had fallen out. In public, she sometimes wore a pale blue bandanna knotted at the back of her head. The TV cameras trolling the audiences at the conference sessions for the nightly news report often lingered on Nicole, snagged by her haunting beauty, her intensity of expression as she listened. She was trolling too, for nuggets of fact in the swirling murk of theories. Why had she gotten breast cancer? What were the best treatments?

We had dinner one evening, away from the bustle of the conference, and talked into the night. Nicole mused about the colossal chasm between understanding breast cancer as a doctor and experiencing it as a patient. Two different worlds. Could the twain meet? I thought so, with a special kind of person, one who could slide the two lenses into one focus, like a stereoscope you slide slowly down the track until the image springs into clarity. A person like Nicole.

"When I had my breast cancer diagnosis and consulted with you at the Wakefield Clinic, Nicole," one of her patients later wrote to her, "I remember how wonderfully helpful you were, sharing with me the wisdom of your experience and your expertise. You made me feel that this was something that *could* be dealt with. You exuded confidence and determination, and it was infectious because I put behind me any thought that this thing could not be beaten. . . ."

Another wrote: "I've extolled your prowess as the best doctor I've ever had in far corners of the world on a recent trip."

It was this dual role of patient-physician, however, that caused such devastation for Nicole later.

Over dinner that night in Kingston, we talked about family, about our kids, about what happens when life suddenly turns and kicks you in the teeth. And we laughed a lot, because how else do you deal with such a blow? You could whine and whimper, you could lie down on the mat and wait for the referee to count to 10 so you could throw in the towel. But Nicole was not a whiner or whimperer. She was a doer, and a fighter. But we did ask, "Why us?"

We came to understand that the only real answer to this question is, "Why *not* us?" A logical response maybe, clever, tidy and fitting in the world of philosophy or logic, even in a generic discussion of disease, but totally useless when it's your body that cancer seems to be devouring. We weren't feeling particularly logical or philosophical or even very scientific that night. At that point we were less interested in what exactly breast cancer was—Nicole would have known certainly, and I just knew it was a very bad thing to have—we just wanted to know, what had we done to get it? What had our bodies done, our cells, our genes, our forebears? What had we eaten, or not eaten; what had we breathed or not breathed? Was it because of stress? Did we have "cancer personalities," our suppressed anger coagulating into tumours? Was it because of weak immune systems? Was it because of bad physiology, bad timing, bad karma, or just plain bad luck?

Some experts theorize that we all have cancer cells in our bodies all the time, but strong immune systems keep them under control. If so, what galvanized our scatter of submissive cells into an unruly legion on the march? Only two years earlier, researchers had found two genes they were sure were the answer. Mutations in these genes were thought to cause normal cells to go haywire, multiplying like young hoods on the mean streets, terrorizing the town. What set our cell gangs roaming the innocent suburban neighbourhoods of our bodies? Was it an inherited mutation or did some environmental factor nudge one of these genes into transmitting garbled instructions to the cells, causing really bad behaviour?

Sherwin Nuland, author and clinical professor of surgery at Yale University School of Medicine, calls cancer cells the "juvenile delinquents of cellular society." "In the community of living tissues, the uncontrolled mob of misfits that is cancer behaves like a gang of perpetually wilding adolescents."[2] Nicole's oncologist also referred to cancer cells as unruly teenage gangs, oddly whimsical language for a scientist. So unfathomable is the source of cancer and so unpredictable its behaviour, perhaps the only accurate way of expressing its awful mystery is through metaphor.

We were keen to know what was the tipping point in our own breast cancer outbreak. Was it like the Hush Puppies epidemic? In the 1990s, a few teenage anti-fashionistas in New York started to wear Hush Puppies, a move that transformed into a movement that swelled into what many viewed as a fashion plague of unlovely footwear across North America. And it did so for no apparent reason. Same with our cancer cells. In the Hush Puppies epidemic, three elements were at play: contagiousness, the fact that little causes have big effects and change occurring not gradually but at one dramatic moment.[3] These are the elements of all epidemics. It felt to us that we each had our own internal private epidemic—a few cancer cells multiplying (contagion), the transformation of a few harmless cells into a very harmful tumour (little causes with big effects) and the one dramatic moment when this happened. But who knew? We did know the tipping point in our conscious lives, that shattering moment when we were told that we had breast cancer. But the tipping point at the cellular level was shrouded in secret, a stealthy flip when everything changed all at once. What had transformed our normal, well-behaved cells into monster children? How could we bring them back under control? Just how did we get into this other place anyway, and how could we get out alive?

⤫

When you are told you have breast cancer, your life tends to fall apart. For that moment, and many after, you rocket through a mine-field of emotions as you come to terms with what you perceive as nothing less than a death sentence. And most people experience them all to some degree: explosions of terror, depression, anger, resignation, fear—sometimes contained in the daylight, but raging out of control in the dark—bitterness, determination, cynicism, pessimism, optimism, black humour, terror again . . . You dance or crawl through the aftermath of the initial strike, blinded by the smoke, ears ringing with the doctor's words, "Yes, it is breast cancer." How the message is delivered—whether gently, peremptorily, in person, by phone—is not what matters. It is the words themselves that cleave your soul. Later you perhaps start parsing their delivery.

When you start to see again, hear again, that's when you begin to notice that breast cancer the disease has not slouched alone into your life. You'll see that it is dragging with it a clanking sack of accessories, a rattle bag of issues that accompanies any disease we don't know enough about, such as what causes it, who it will strike, who it will kill, who it will savage and then let go, and what will cure it. So as well as struggling with the physical disease, with the knowledge that malevolent cells are running rampant within your body, you get to struggle with the baggage breast cancer brings with it.

First out of the rattle bag is the question of cause, paramount because until we know for certain what causes breast cancer, we won't know with any certainty what will cure or prevent it. This is a harsh reality for researchers who see progress in the labs wither in the wards, for doctors trying to cure or control the disease, and for decision makers trying to set policy. It is harshest of all for someone newly diagnosed who discovers that no one has the answers to her question, What caused my cancer? When you go searching, you end up not with certainties but in a tangle of myth, theories debunked and reinstated and debunked again, and risk factors, those confusing, shifting, contentious and often dangerous prescriptives that elbow each other for supremacy in your new world. All these sit somewhere on the cause continuum.

Superficially, the notion of causality *seems* straightforward: you have a cause and you have an effect, or rather, you have a continuum—a cause leading to a cause leading to a cause leading to another cause, until you have, in effect, a river of causes. Dipping into that river is like fly fishing in a trout stream. What "cause" you catch depends on where you cast your line, and where you cast your line depends on who you are. A genetic scientist fishes pretty close to where the river rises, and catches a gene. An environmentalist might also catch a gene but is more interested in grasping whatever caused that gene to be in the river in the first place. Physicians follow a selective catch-and-release program, their decision to keep or reject the fish as cause/risk factor/myth dictated by the latest research. And women newly diagnosed with breast cancer probably aren't fishing from the river's banks at all but floundering neck deep in it, trying to keep from drowning.

The river metaphor may illustrate the various levels of cause but it doesn't truly reflect the complexity of causality in breast cancer—all the causal loops. "You think it should be linear, you think it should be 'A' to 'B' and then 'B' to 'C' and 'C' to 'D,'" Scott Findlay says. "But that's not how it works. It's 'A' to 'B, C, D, E,' then it's 'B' to 'E, D, C and F,' etc., etc.; it's this whole network going on."[4] More like a vat of alphabet soup than a river.

A true cause is something that is necessary and sufficient to make another event happen. "Necessary and sufficient" is the pivotal phrase. You can have necessary but not sufficient. Or sufficient but not necessary. Both are needed for it to be a bona fide cause. When I first heard this definition, I thought it was scientific doublespeak; I couldn't grasp the simplicity of the concept. But it is the clearest, cleanest, most elegant definition of cause, the litmus test that separates risk factors from causes. Scott, a biologist, uses the "green lake" example to explain the concept: "I have a lake. I throw a bunch of phosphorous in the lake and the lake becomes green. This is repeatable. Whenever I throw phosphorous into any lake, it will go green, so it is a *sufficient* cause. It is not a *necessary* cause though, because other things can turn a lake green. However, if I throw phosphorous in a lake and it turns green, and nothing else can turn a lake green, then phosphorous is also a *necessary* cause."

You can use this formula to try and establish whether something causes cancer, for example, the BRCA genes, which, when first discovered, were thought to be where breast cancer started. If mutations in these two genes were a necessary cause, then every woman with breast cancer would have the mutations; if they were a sufficient cause, then all women with the mutations would have breast cancer. This, however, is not the case. Less than 10 percent of women with breast cancer have one or both of these genes. So clearly, the BRCA1 and BRCA2 mutations are neither "necessary" nor "sufficient" for breast cancer. This, in a nutshell, is the difference between risk factor and cause. The presence of both conditions establishes a cause, the presence of one or the other suggests a risk factor, and the presence of neither suggests you might be dealing with myth.

THE DANGER OF MYTHS

Myths are the bottom-feeders in the causal river, surfacing from the murk to scare women unnecessarily in a world where there are enough real things to worry about. These are the stories you hear that build from idle surmise to "scientifically proven fact" but are really nothing more than the end result of a more widespread and pernicious version of the children's game Pass the Word. These stories don't belong in the risk factor category at all but cling like catfish to the rumours and bad data that spawn them.

Mythical "causes" of breast cancer are exploded regularly yet stitch themselves back together to rise phoenix-like from the studies that have debunked them. For example, there is the notion that deodorants cause breast cancer. No they don't. It is thought that one widely distributed anonymous e-mail gave wings to this myth. It caused enough angst that such august organizations as the American Cancer Society and the US-based National Cancer Institute issued statements refuting the claim, and researchers took it seriously enough to submit the theory to controlled studies. Most recent, at the time of writing, was one study conducted by epidemiologists at the Fred Hutchinson

Cancer Research Center in Seattle that found no link between the disease and deodorant.[5] That is certainly not the end of it, though. Deodorants continue to be described as a possible cause in the less reputable "health" literature you often see in the local supermarket.

You might also hear that you caused your breast cancer by dyeing your hair. No you didn't. A study published in the *European Journal of Cancer* in September 2002 found no difference in the "hair colouring practices" of 608 women who had been diagnosed with and treated for breast cancer and 609 similarly aged healthy women.[6]

Such studies should blow these myths out of the water but don't because the free-floating fear of breast cancer will snag on just about any possible "cause," no matter how loony. Other items that have endured on the mythical list of breast cancer causes are:

- coffee (although this one is slipping down the charts, and a recent study even indicates that caffeine might actually lower risk, at least for skin cancer in hairless mice. Lab mice slathered with caffeine developed fewer skin tumours than—uh—decaffeinated animals.)[7]
- synthetic bras
- large breasts
- wet ear wax
- scented soap
- living under hydro wires
- not enough sunlight
- too much sunlight
- breast-feeding
- not breast-feeding

The list goes on. The Canadian Cancer Society website now includes a sensible and reassuring discussion of the major "cancer myths" that is worth checking out. (www.cancer.ca/ccs/)

One item that, for the moment, has bounced out of the myth category and into the possible risk factor zone is exposure to too much nocturnal light. Some research indicates that the proliferation of bedroom night lights, street lights and headlights confuse our circadian rhythms and interfere with our bodies' ability to produce melatonin— a cancer-inhibiting hormone the body produces mainly at night. The Harvard University's Nurses' Health Study found a 40 percent increase in breast cancer risk among shift workers who are constantly subjected to artificial light.[8]

Some claims that swing back and forth between myth and risk factor category actually achieve the status of direct cause in some circles. These claims are tougher to deal with because their link with mainstream research, however spurious, lends them an air of credibility and because they carry with them a moral big stick with which to hammer in the guilt. You hear, like whispered gossip in a village tea room, that abortions cause breast cancer, or at least are a risk factor. They don't and they aren't, according to a consensus of experts and reputable studies. The claim allegedly originated with two anti-abortionists, Joel Brind, a New York science teacher, and Scott Somerville, a lawyer with no scientific or medical training, who says: "'To understand the biological mechanism, you don't have to be a brain surgeon. When a pregnancy is ended prematurely by an abortion or miscarriage, the hormonal changes that swell a women's breasts and prepare her for pregnancy are interrupted. The cells in the breast never complete the process of differentiation and specialization, leaving them immature and more susceptible to carcinogens.'"[9]

The Coalition on Abortion/Breast Cancer claims that "28 out of 37 studies in the world-wide literature" indicate that induced abortions increase the risk of breast cancer. Spontaneous abortions apparently don't, "having no significant effect on risks."[10] It is not explained why a spontaneous abortion or miscarriage does not interrupt cell development in the same way as an induced abortion allegedly does.

Alarmed by such claims based on what it sees as misinterpretation and manipulation of data, the American Cancer Society got into a legal tussle with the Coalition over its misuse of the Society's own research, resulting in the Coalition's following call to arms:

After 44 years of published studies on the abortion-breast cancer research, it has become very apparent that the powers-that-be do not intend to share this information with the public. . . . The only way that women will be told the truth is if individuals who are aware of the research take this matter into their own hands to make it a grass-roots movement. Those who have knowledge of the abortion-breast cancer research are morally obligated to share the information with friends, relatives and neighbors and for doing everything possible, within their means, to spread the word within their communities.[11]

To try to stem such a "morally obligated" spreading of the word, the Canadian Cancer Society, in September 2002, published its official position on the issue:

Current scientific evidence does not support a relationship between abortion and any type of breast cancer in women with or without a family history of cancer. . . . Although some studies have shown slightly increased risk of breast cancer in relation to induced abortion, many of these studies have substantial weaknesses. In fact, the strongest studies show no relationship whatsoever between abortion and breast cancer.[12]

It would be good if we could leave the myths and misconceptions buried in the silt at the bottom of the river, but unfortunately they have a relentless buoyancy that keeps them in circulation. It would be even better if everyone agreed on what is a myth and what is a credible risk factor. That will happen only when we know exactly what the underlying cause(s) of breast cancer are.

THE RISK OF RISK FACTORS

When you look up "risk factor" in the index of the *Cancer Dictionary,* you will find more than 80 entries, ranging from albinism to X-rays.[13] Of course, these are not all for breast cancer; in fact, most of the ones specific to breast cancer aren't even included, but it gives you a sense of just how risky it is out there. Some risk factors are avoidable, or controllable by you, as much of the literature tells you—smoking is invariably the example used—but many are not. Eating and breathing, for instance.

It's hard to know how to deal with risk factors. You might be fatalistic and assume that breast cancer is either written on your forehead or not, and assume that whatever happens was destined to happen. Or you can be proactive and try to dodge at least the avoidable risk factors. There is an old joke about the River Liffey that flows through Dublin, a river, despite its majesty and charm, of effluence and sludge. A fellow on the quay asks his companion in disbelief, "Look, that's never someone swimming out there, is it?" His friend peers through the steam rising off the polluted water, and replies, "Ah, not at all, he's just going through the motions." Sometimes that's what it feels like; you can spend a lot of energy ducking and bobbing in the headwaters of possible risk factors that might have no link to cancer at all.

A risk factor is "a substance or condition that increases the chance of developing a particular cancer. . . . The degree of risk each factor poses depends on a number of different things and can vary from person to person."[14] It can be seen as a contributing cause, but it's not the underlying cause. It is established through statistical analysis of correlation, rather than on any firm understanding of how it might result in the formation of breast cancer cells. Correlation is not cause, but to date it's all we've got.

Ubiquitous as loosestrife, risk factors guide much of the research; they are listed in most articles on breast cancer published in the popular media; they grace the pamphlets and handouts from breast cancer organizations; they are the subject of sessions at conferences; and they twist our lives into pretzels when we interpret them as causes and try to live by them. They have evolved into rules of conduct, many of which we cannot live by, and many of which we shouldn't live by, especially since the rules keep changing.

Many of the current risk factors are enduring, anointed by science, consensus and history. They have appeared on the Top 10 risk list for centuries, first as causes, often without any understanding of why they should be linked with the disease, then as factors having a close correlation with breast cancer. With the convergence of conjecture and science in the decades following the Second World War, they were given new legs and resurfaced in more sophisticated garb provided by labs and statistics. Advances in scientific knowledge have shifted them from the realm of surmise to a much more credible footing, though as contributing factors rather than as causes.

As early as 1700, the "female factor" was observed by the Italian physician Bernardino Ramazzini, who noticed an unusually high incidence of breast cancer among nuns. "You seldom find," he wrote, "a convent that does not harbor this accursed pest, cancer, within its walls."[15] In the 1800s, a study in Italy showed that nuns were almost 10 times more likely to die of breast cancer than from uterine cancer.[16] These centuries-old observations have found footing in current research suggesting that prolonged exposure to hormonal activity because of early menarche and late menopause, or the years of reproductive life uninterrupted by pregnancies, increases the risk of genetic damage and can result in breast cancer.

The same Ramazzini was one of the first to make the connection between cancer and environmental causes when he observed that workers in particular occupations were especially prone to cancer: "'Various and manifold . . . is the harvest of diseases reaped by certain workers from the crafts they pursue. All the profit that they get is fatal injury to their health.'"[17] In 1775, an English doctor, Percival Pott, made the first recorded connection between cancer and a specific external irritant, claiming that repeated exposure to soot gave chimney sweeps cancer of the scrotum, called "soot-wart" then, "squamous cell carcinoma" now. Epidemiologists in the 1880s reported a large number of lung cancers among miners in Germany: "This was the first clear record . . . of an internal neoplasm [new growth or cancer] being caused by an environmental exposure to a complex carcinogen."[18] It wasn't until the genetic discoveries of the 20th century that these connections were understood—that an "irritant" such as tobacco or coal dust or coal tar could damage a gene, unleashing the "teenage gangs" of cancer cells.

I'm not sure when "risk factors" came into common usage, but you find the term scattered through much of the popular literature as far back as 30 years ago. A book published in 1974 and distributed free as a "for the public good" gesture by one of the big American book clubs features many of the same risk factors as today: "Age . . . plays an important role. Breast cancer is primarily a disease of mature women. . . . A woman who has her first full-term baby before the age of 20 has her risk of developing breast cancer reduced by two thirds. . . . A first, full-term birth when the mother is past 30 seems to increase the risk of breast cancer. . . . An interesting relationship exists between frequency of breast cancer and the age of onset of menstruation and the age at menopause. . . . In general, the more years of menstrual activity, the greater likelihood for breast cancer to develop."[19]

Thirty-five years later, the same factors are present, expressed with slightly more scientific certainty, but with little progress attendant in how to deal with them. At the Third World Conference on Breast Cancer in Victoria, B.C., the hormone effect, aging and family history of breast cancer were presented almost as if the connections were newly established. The only apparent difference was the rather desperate shift in responsibility for dealing with them.

The current risk factors associated with the development of breast cancer are:

- Aging
- Having had breast cancer before
- Genetic factors: having a mother or sister who has had the disease, or an otherwise strong history of breast cancer in the family

- Hormonal factors: never having children; not having a first full-term pregnancy until after the age of 30; having had early onset of menstruation, before 12 years of age, or late onset of menopause, after 55 years of age; having been on hormone replacement therapy (HRT) for more than five years. Dr. Katherine Wynne-Edwards of Queen's University says there is a 120-fold increase in risk associated with modern lifestyle but zeros in on estrogen exposure in particular: "I'm not saying that estrogen is causing breast cancer, but I'm saying it's in the room, around the corner and facilitating breast cancer." Definitely one of the black cats in the dark room. Wynne-Edwards has launched a study called Daughters without Breast Cancer to measure the estrogen levels in the saliva of 3,000 girls across Canada between the ages of 9 and 17. "I'm asking them to spit for science and put it in the home freezer."[20]
- Having had two or more breast biopsies for benign conditions, or experiencing changes in the breasts such as atypical hyperplasia (abnormal cell growth causing enlargement of tissues) or lobular carcinoma in situ (tiny cancers confined to the lobules of the breast)
- A high-fat/low-fibre diet
- No or low physical exercise
- Being obese, especially in the post-menopausal years. Research findings published in May 2003 found that obesity is "a significant risk factor for death from cancer." Out of just over 900,000 adults in the United States who were cancer free at enrolment in the study, 57,245 died of cancer during the 16-year follow-up. "The heaviest members of this cohort"—those with a body-mass index of at least 40—had a death rate 52 percent higher (for men) and 62 percent higher (for women) than those of normal weight. Breast cancer was high on the list of cancers in which this trend showed up.[21]
- Smoking. In the space of four years, smoking went from a possible *prevention* factor for developing breast cancer to a major

risk factor: a 1998 study suggested that the risk of breast cancer for women who carry the mutation in the BRCA1 or BRCA2 genes might be decreased by cigarette smoking.[22] Three years later, other researchers found that smoking significantly increases the risk of breast cancer for women with a strong family history of the disease.[23] Then a clear link was found between smoking and breast cancer among women without any other risk factors,[24] and two months later, Canadian researchers found that teenage girls almost double their risk of getting breast cancer if they start smoking within five years of their first menstrual period. Even if they quit in their early 20s, the damage may already have been done.[25]

- Using alcohol excessively. This factor has been on and off the list like a jumping-bean, but recent studies put it back on because of the interaction between alcohol consumption and estrogen. Although estrogen is synthesized and secreted by the ovaries, it is metabolized for use by the liver. It has been found that the liver cells in some women are hypersensitive to alcohol, and this may allow increased levels of estrogen to remain in the blood. The hormone could then influence cells that have already undergone an early premalignant change.[26] However, at a recent conference on breast cancer, back-to-back presentations by two doctors offered opposing views: one doctor from Australia advised that drinking stouts and wines in moderation was a good thing; another advised total abstinence, a view supported by at least one new study published in 2008 (see introduction).
- Having over 75 percent dense breast tissue (if the tissue is mostly glandular tissue), especially in women who are at least 45 years of age
- Iatrogenic factors (caused by treatment itself), such as previous radiation therapy for childhood cancers such as Hodgkin's disease or leukemia
- Living in North America or western Europe
- Exposure to environmental toxins

It would follow, then, that a 55-year-old, obese, heavy-smoking, hard-drinking, Caucasian nun living, but never exercising, in North America, with a prolonged menopausal history, whose mother and sister had premenopausal bilateral breast cancer, who has had breast cancer before, who has had radiation treatments for childhood leukemia, who breathed DDT as a child wouldn't stand a chance.[27]

The thing is, even that woman might never get breast cancer—or might get it once but then not again—and the young Asian woman living down the street, recently arrived from Japan who runs to work, who is vegetarian and eats only organic foods, who had her first baby at age 15, who has never smoked, who drinks only spring water might. (Incidence of breast cancer among Asian women is comparatively low until they emigrate to a Western country, but within a generation, the incidence among their population equals that of their adopted country.)

Nicole was 37 when she was diagnosed, so aging did not figure; she exercised regularly, she ate healthily, she did not smoke, so her lifestyle choices did not figure; she did not have either BRCA1 or BRCA2 mutations; her mother and sister did not have breast cancer, nor was there any other strong family history of the disease, so apparently genetics didn't figure; she hadn't had breast cancer before nor had she been treated for any other type of cancer before; she did not have early menarche; she had three children; she was never on HRT—never mind that her menopause was very early, brought on artificially by treatment related to her disease. According to the above list, she shouldn't have gotten breast cancer.

Breast cancer can attack anyone, including men. Men account for about 1 percent of breast cancer cases, and of all the groups with the disease must feel the most marginalized. (For a session on male breast cancer at the 2002 Third World Conference on Breast Cancer, an audience of about 30 people, including a handful of men, showed up—but the presenter didn't.) And they don't get much of a look-in with many of the risk factors, particularly the main one—being female.

The startling fact is that, in most cases, breast cancer hits women who are not classified as high risk: 75 percent of women with the disease have no other risk factors than that they *are* women. This is the kicker in confusing risk factor with cause. We crunch the cause continuum, telescope the stages, replace "risk" with "cause" and come up with a rule such as, "If you smoke, you'll get cancer." Not necessarily. Lots of people smoke but don't get cancer. Not every chimney sweep got scrotum cancer; not everyone dies of cancer if he or she lives to be 85; not everyone who has a mutated BRCA1 or BRCA2 gene gets breast cancer. Correlation might plot a path of increased risk, but not one of direct cause.

It's not just the media, or cancer patients themselves, who interchange the term "risk " with "cause." Even scientists sometimes flip these terms, and when they do, the confusion deepens even more. You think you've just got it straight, you grasp that nobody knows what actually causes cancer and then you read in a prestigious scientific tome on risk assessment that "major *causes* [my emphasis] of cancer are: (1) smoking, which accounts for 31 percent of US cancer deaths and 87 percent of lung cancer deaths, (2) dietary imbalances, which account for about another third (e.g., lack of sufficient amounts of dietary fruits and vegetables), (3) chronic infections, mostly in developing countries, and (4) hormonal factors, which are influenced primarily by lifestyle."[28]

Not only are these not causes, but these scientists throw a curveball by suggesting that hormonal factors are lifestyle choices. Women are good, women are great, but even women can't choose whether to be born female, or when to start their periods. (Up until late 2002, we were encouraged to think that, by using HRT, we could effectively control when our periods ended, but this has turned out to be not the attractive choice we thought it was these last 20 years. A huge hormone replacement study was abruptly halted that year because it found that women on estrogen and progestin for more than five years had a 26 percent higher risk of developing breast cancer than women who did not take HRT.)

The persistent misuse of the term "risk factor" can have an enormously damaging impact on women's lives. We seem to keep forgetting, despite it being implicit in the definition of "risk factors," that the degree of their impact depends on a number of different things and can vary from person to person. This is not just a game in semantics: it is the breeding ground for misunderstandings of a magnitude that makes this disease harder to understand, and harder to bear. The woolly thinking that confuses "risk factor" with "cause" has led to untold misery; it has given rise to the hoary spectre of guilt and blame-the-victim syndrome. Most damaging is its insidious influence on treatment decisions.

First the guilt. In response to a question about whether he thought there had been progress over the last 30 years in breast cancer treatment, one cancer surgeon I spoke to responded this way: "Oh yes. First of all I think there is a lot more awareness out there; there are a lot of great programs to disseminate information and make women aware of their responsibility towards their own health and in particular their own breast health. This leads obviously to an earlier diagnosis, and with an early diagnosis we are hopefully going to find smaller tumours, less aggressive tumours, [so that] long-term outcome will be improved." The "progress" this surgeon sees is in increased patient or potential-patient responsibility for making sure they don't get the disease in the first place. And if they do, for making sure they find it early so that the tools doctors do have to treat the disease might have a chance of working.

You can see what a minefield this is—how easy it is for women to feel they are to blame for getting breast cancer. Linda Varner, the breast cancer patient coordinator at the Dr. Léon Richard Oncology Centre in Moncton, New Brunswick, says this is one of the most common and distressing of concerns: "Women ask me, 'What caused my breast cancer?' I get this question all the time. They are in shock and disbelief. They say, 'I did everything right, I never smoked, I ate healthily, I exercised.' They feel they have done something wrong. [It is hard for them to understand that] risk factors are just about the *possibilities* of getting breast cancer."[29] The danger lies not in risk factors themselves, but in our perception of them. When a woman applies an individual risk factor to her own situation, it can skewer her with guilt or helplessness.

More pernicious still is the influence these misconceptions have on physicians' advice and on women's decisions about preventative treatment. Many women who have been deemed high risk for getting breast cancer, based on assessments of the latest risk factor research, choose to have a prophylactic mastectomy (breast removal to try to prevent cancer) or an oophorectomy (surgical removal of the ovaries to reduce hormonal activity), even though they do not have breast cancer. They are just so afraid they might get it. Researchers at the University of Toronto found that almost a quarter of women who had chosen to have their breasts removed to prevent cancer had overestimated their risk of developing the disease. Researchers Steven Narod and Kelly Metcalfe say that a likely explanation for the decision to take such a radical step was "cancer worry," which is more closely linked to perceived risk than to actual risk. "We don't know what is driving these perceptions, whether it's from the media, their families or physicians. But it is troubling."[30]

You bet it's troubling. It's not difficult to trace the source of cancer worry experienced by women: the trail leads straight to risk factors, and women's misconceptions of risk, and to the shifting bulletins from the research world that constantly recalibrate risk according to the latest study. In the context of science, such research is progress, even if studies disagree with each other. In the context of the reality of women's lives, the conflicting data are confusing and can be truly destructive if used as a foundation for personal treatment decisions.

It is a difficult situation for doctors as well. Dr. Shail Verma, an oncologist who runs a high-risk clinic at the Ottawa Regional Cancer Centre, says, "There is no clear route for high-risk women. . . . We can't keep having women come to a high-risk clinic just to be told they are high risk, but we have no answers yet."[31]

The choices are just as fraught, and the outcomes equally uncertain, for women who have had breast cancer and decide on prophylactic surgery to try to head off recurrence. Following her treatment for primary cancer—cancer contained within the breast—Nicole elected to have a second mastectomy mainly because she hated the feeling of lopsidedness caused by her first mastectomy. She also wanted to slam as many doors as possible against recurrence. This extreme decision was based on her own professional assessment of the current research, as well as her doctor's. It was not an easy decision to make, nor was it based on a misinterpretation of risk assessment. Her cancer came back anyway.

Information pours in from genetic researchers, and like weather predictions, some models shift risk status from hurricanes, to gales, to strong winds; others ratchet the risk back up to hurricane status. Researchers face the overwhelming task of mapping, processing and analyzing the million data points pouring out of genome research. Women are buffeted by the shifting statistics they need to make crucial, life-altering decisions. Do they batten down the hatches and keep sailing? Do they opt for drastic prophylactic measures—bilateral mastectomies and oophorectomies—to weather a storm that might never materialize? The one choice they don't have is not to sail at all. The researchers will continue to issue their forecasts based on the current and best data, and women must either continue to steer a course dictated by these forecasts or ignore them completely and hope that the storm doesn't break.

What should you do about risk factors if you, understandably, suffer from cancer worry? Put them at the bottom of your worry list. It is useless to fret about the ones you can't do anything about (being a woman, growing old or having the wrong genes) and equally unproductive to feel guilty about some of the others, such as "wrong" lifestyle choices (since many women who have made the same choices never get breast cancer).

Nevertheless, until research determines the causes of breast cancer, we must make do with risk factors. The controversies and disagreements will continue because risk factors shift, shedding or taking on certainty with each new wave of research. They will leap on and off the latest "definitive" list like fleas. Yet they are necessary evils, like an amorphous, unpredictable crowd of guides—some reliable, some fraudulent and chimeric—on the cause continuum.

On its website, the American Cancer Society states: "Although we know some of the risk factors that increase a woman's chance of developing breast cancer, we do not yet know what causes most breast cancers or exactly how some of these risk factors cause cells to become cancerous. Research is under way to learn more."[32] There is a kind of despairing honesty in these words, but they about sum up the current situation.

2 SEARCHING FOR THE BLACK BOX: THE GENE STORY

*The notion of causality in general in science is like quicksilver:
you try to grab it and it disappears. With cancer, you have
a web of causality—you have the proximate cause and
the ultimate cause and you have everything in between.*

—Scott Findlay, biologist[1]

MADELEINE H. has lived all her life in Bathurst, New Brunswick.
When I met her, she was staying at a residential oncology centre in
Moncton for treatment for a second bout of breast cancer. She'd
already had one mastectomy, she'd taken tamoxifen (a hormone
therapy) for five years, and here came the cancer again. A purple
grid—like a bad tattoo—glowed on her neck above her collar, indicating the target area for her radiation.

The centre was too far away for her to commute each day—it was a
three-and-a-half-hour drive from Bathurst—so she lived there for five
days each week, separated from her family and friends. She was lucky, she
said, to have such a pleasant place to stay. And it was. Light and airy, with

plump chintz-covered sofas in a softly elegant common room, full of sun that day, with flowers on the blond wood coffee table in front of us.

A map of New Brunswick hangs in the hallway, studded with coloured pins indicating where patients at the centre have come from. The North Shore bears a solid line of pins. This could mean that there is a greater concentration of population there, therefore more patients. Or it could mean that the incidence of cancer is actually higher in that area. Most of the people I spoke to in Moncton believed that was likely the case. The industrial North Shore is speckled with mines and mills that for decades have spewed toxins into the air and water of the region.

Madeleine spoke quietly and matter-of-factly about the cancer that has torn through her family. Female relatives had mastectomies almost as often as they had babies: "My two sisters both have had breast cancer; they're both younger than me. One had a mastectomy almost 20 years ago; she had her second one about a month ago. She was down this week to see the oncologist and now she has to have chemo. She has a more aggressive form of cancer this time. My other sister, she's 10 years younger than I am—she had her breast removed last year. . . .

"My mother had breast cancer but when she was an old lady. It didn't kill her though—she died of other things. My father's sister had breast cancer . . . so I guess I am a good candidate."[2]

Madeleine had already had cancer of the cervix when she found the first lump in her breast. "I knew exactly what it was. I wasn't surprised. You have to take things as they come." She laughs. "There's not much you can do about it. You just get rid of one thing and go on to the next."

Cancer, she meant. You get rid of one cancer and go on to the next cancer. It seemed that she and her sisters parcelled the years of their lives between cancer recurrences.

When I asked her what she thought caused all that cancer, she smiled with resignation. "I guess it's a combination of the genes and the mills," she said. The genes and the mills. What a team.

The earliest theories of what causes breast cancer were embedded in mythology; the current theories are embedded in science. Mystery still accompanies them all. The Greek physician Hippocrates, considered to be the father of medicine, postulated that disease was caused by an imbalance of the four humours—blood, phlegm, yellow bile and black bile—normally kept stable by natural forces in the body. When the four humours are balanced, we are healthy. When they get out of whack, we are sick. If Nicole and Madeleine and I had been living during Hippocrates' lifetime (about 460 to 377 B.C., but history is hazy), we'd have been told that our tumours were the result of abnormal humoral accretions.

The attribution of causation to something physical rather than supernatural was a big step in medical understanding. Until then, illness and disease were considered to be the mysterious handiwork of the gods. In the second century A.D., the Greek physician Galen of Pergamon believed that cancer was an infection caused by a flux of black bile and an excess of blood flowing through the veins. Versions of the humoral theory of disease that had black bile roaring through our arterial systems like a tsunami of cancer held sway for 1,400 years. Vestiges of it hung about even into the 19th century.

In the 1700s, it was thought that cancer was caused by coagulating lymph (the fluid that carries white blood cells through the lymph system); this belief that the lymph system was actually a causal factor in the spread of cancer rather than simply a conduit for cancer cells to travel to other parts of the body persisted until the 1970s.

In the 19th century, German pathologist Rudolf Virchow discovered that diseases came from abnormal changes within already existing cells; abnormal cells multiplied through division, resulting in tumours. This was a huge leap in the understanding of cancer pathology because until then cancer had been considered a mysteriously systemic disorder that did not have a localized source, and so defied containment.

A countervailing theory during the latter half of the 19th century was that disease was caused by germs. The two theories, both enormously significant developments, fought for supremacy as researchers and physicians tried to apply one or the other to all disease. The proponents of the germ theory posited that if cancer was caused by a germ, it must mean it was contagious, a view held by many into the 20th century. In 1913, when a guest died of cancer in his hotel, a Swiss hotelkeeper, "sure that cancer germs were spreading through his establishment, destroyed the bedroom furniture and sued the widow for $255 in damages."[3]

History is littered with unusual causal theories about cancer. Like trout. Around 1910, US President William Howard Taft was so convinced that trout were at the root of all cancer that he asked Congress to appropriate $50,000 to support the relevant research. Congress turned him down. The director of the New York State Institute for the Study of Malignant Disease, however, agreed with him: It was an astonishing coincidence, he said, "'that the distribution of this variety of fish and the concentration of cancer in man in this country are almost identical. A map of one might well be taken as a map of the other.'"[4] The *New York Times* agreed, saying that the president's proposal was "the greatest stroke so far toward the conquest of the dread disease. . . ."[5]

The cancer by trauma theory—that a local irritation, a bump or bruise, could cause cancer—was widely accepted in the first half of the 20th century, when it was estimated by some that trauma was responsible for 50 percent of bone cancers.[6]

In 1949, Anita Menarde fell getting off a Philadelphia streetcar and was treated for a bruised ankle and knee and scraped hands. That night she noticed a discolouration on her right side and breast. Her doctor prescribed hot compresses, and for two months all was well. Then she found a lump, which was diagnosed as cancerous; she sued the Philadelphia streetcar company for causing her cancer and won. In 1964, a woman bruised her breast and broke her leg in a store, developed breast cancer 14 months later and sued the store owners. "One physician discerned a connection [between her fall and breast cancer], six did not, and the jury awarded her $40,000."[7]

The cancer by trauma theory lingers. In many developing countries, a commonly held belief is that breast cancer can be caused by the bump of an infant's head while nursing.

In 1915, two Japanese researchers discovered that by painting rabbits' ears with tar, they could cause cancer, confirming what many researchers had been saying for centuries, that man-made chemicals were implicated in the disease. It would have been difficult to know, without 21st-century hindsight, which discovery was the more important in cancer research—that we could cause cancers in the lab, on purpose, or that we were causing cancer, not on purpose, outside it.

If we were searching in the 1940s for answers to why we got cancer, Nicole and I would have learned that it was caused by "civilization, filth, population density, air pollution, diets, sex life, emotional trauma, occupation, geophysical radiation, tea drinking, heredity . . . nerves, social status, injury and chronic irritation."[8] Culled from a literature search of 8,500 articles listed in the Index Catalogue of the US Surgeon General's Office published between 1923 and 1938, these hypotheses were the ones most commonly held at that time. Seven decades later, with the addition of scientific underpinnings and the use of different terminology, most still are.

The Second World War unleashed a torrent of science, originally to further military ends, but at the end of the conflict, science was put to use in other areas, particularly medicine. In the United States, grants doled out to the National Institutes of Health jumped from $180,000 in the fiscal year 1945 to $4 million in 1947. That same year, the National Cancer Institute of Canada was born as a joint initiative of the Department of National Health and Welfare and the Canadian Cancer Society. Its mandate was to coordinate efforts to reduce the morbidity and mortality from cancer by supporting clinical and laboratory-based research.

Exposure to radiation became a focus of attention in relation to increased breast cancer incidence following the hydrogen bomb tests in the 1950s and 1960s, 90 of which were carried out between 1952 and 1957 at the Nevada Test Site alone. These explosions blanketed the continent, and when "fallout from all tests, domestic and foreign, is taken together, no U.S. [and, it follows, Canadian] resident born after 1951 escaped exposure." It is estimated that about 22,000 cancers were the result, from "melanoma to breast cancer."[9] Researchers working on the Atomic Bomb Study reported: "At this point, there can be little doubt that radiation exposure of breast tissue during infancy and early childhood could contribute to the risk of breast cancer during adult life."[10]

Rosalie Bertell, a highly respected activist, founder and immediate past president of the International Institute of Concern for Public Health in Toronto, agrees. Nicole and I heard her speak at the First World Conference on Breast Cancer in Kingston in July of 1997. It was a sobering experience. She said, without mincing words, that radiation is the best documented of all causes of breast cancer.[11]

By now, in our quest for answers to "Why me?" it was beginning to look as though everything caused breast cancer—not a good sign, because the proliferation of theories is usually in direct proportion to how much is not known about a disease. So, when two breast cancer genes were identified in 1994 and 1995, there was great excitement. The black box of breast cancer had been found. Finally, finally, we'd know, clearly, absolutely, what caused our breast cancer. A mutant gene, or two.

James Watson, Nobel laureate and co-discoverer of DNA, referred to the race to isolate the breast cancer gene as "the most exciting story in medical science." It was also one of the most competitive and publicly visible. In October 1990, Dr. Mary-Claire King announced at the annual conference of the American Society of Human Genetics that her team had found evidence of a gene that linked heredity and the risk of breast cancer. The race was on. Scientists in several countries, including Dr. Steven Narod of Canada, were involved in the four-year search, and in September 1994, BRCA1 was identified on chromosome 17 by an American team of researchers led by Mark Skolnick. Soon after, a large collaborative group of researchers from Britain and the United States discovered the location of BRCA2, on chromosome 13, a gene that also implicates breast cancer in men. These discoveries earned headlines around the world.

A "breast cancer gene" is one in which inherited mutations (known as germ-line mutations, as opposed to sporadic mutations, which are not inherited but random) "confer increased susceptibility to breast cancer."[12] Essentially, these genes were identified as "causing" breast cancer because a large proportion of women who had mutations in these genes also had breast cancer. In other words, the relative risk of women with BRCA1 and BRCA2 versus those without is much higher. It is important, though, to recognize that this is a correlation, and like all correlations, does not prove cause. Which helps to explain what happened next.

Within weeks, the researchers found that although the mutant gene apparently "was a major gene in hereditary early-onset breast cancer, it did not appear mutated in the 90 percent or more breast cancers of unknown cause."[13] One scientist said with quiet understatement, "Somewhat disappointingly, follow-up large-scale mutation screening studies determined that not only are BRCA1 and BRCA2 not mutated in sporadic tumours (cancers that arise from an accidental rather than an inherited genetic mutation), but mutations in these two genes are responsible for only a fraction of inherited cases,"[14] now thought to be closer to about 8 percent of all breast cancers.

This obviously was hard luck for women with either of the genes, since it was estimated that they had an 85 percent risk of getting the disease over their lifetime, as compared with 11 percent for other women.[15] It was also hard luck for the remaining 92 percent of women who got breast cancer, because they were still without a clue why they had.

Then in August 2002, a study published in the *Journal of the National Cancer Institute* further rocked the BRCA boat.[16] It suggested that the risk of breast cancer associated with mutations in these two genes appeared to be much lower than previously thought. Estimates of penetrance (the likelihood of a mutation carrier developing breast cancer in her lifetime) were exaggerated because the impact of other risk factors for the disease had not been taken into account—the impact of "nurture" on "nature."

The study's author, Colin Begg, pointed out that "early studies examined families that had multiple cases of breast cancer and resulted in very high penetrance estimates—in the range of 71% to 85% by 70 years of age. . . . More recent studies have used women with breast cancer who do not necessarily have a strong family history of the disease. These studies have resulted in considerably lower estimates."[17]

Another two-edged sword: women who have tested positive for the BRCA genes can take comfort in the new information that their lifetime risk of developing breast cancer has been recalibrated, falling from 85 percent to about 26 percent according to one report.[18] However, this last number is highly contested. Oncologist Shail Verma, who specializes in treating women at high risk for breast cancer, believes that the percentage is probably closer to 50 or 60. But how do women feel who have had, on the basis of the earlier risk estimates, a prophylactic mastectomy or oophorectomy, the recommended treatment of choice up until recently?[19]

Breast cancer genetic researchers must feel that just when they could see light at the end of the tunnel, someone ordered more tunnel. An editorial accompanying Begg's study takes a mildly hectoring tone, saying that it "underscores the pitfalls of failing to address the complexity of disease risk and its implications for disease prevention. . . . Without a healthy respect for the many factors that may influence penetrance, we will continue to overestimate the risk conferred by BRCA1 and BRCA2 mutations alone and, thus, miss opportunities to develop truly effective prevention strategies for women who are genetically susceptible to breast cancer."[20]

The "many factors" might include other low penetrance genes that could make subtle contributions to a person's susceptibility to a disease. Recently, Dutch researchers have identified seven genes responsible for drug resistance and aggressiveness in estrogen-positive breast cancers.[21]

And it seems that non-genetic risk factors—hormonal activity, aging, environmental toxins—can influence the outcome of genetic risk for breast cancer. And stress. Virtually every woman I talked to in researching this book cited stress as the major contributing cause of her cancer.

This is not a new concept. Galen in A.D. 200 noted that cancer was on the increase among "melancholy" women (*melan chole* means "black bile" in Greek). In 1826, Sir Astley Cooper claimed that breast cancer evolved from grief or anxiety, and a few years later the eminent British authority Walter Walsh wrote that cancer often derived from the "influence of mental misery, sudden reverses of fortune, and habitual gloomings of the temper."[22]

Susan Love, author of the bible of breast cancer, *The Susan Love Breast Book,* said she was appalled by a 1984 survey indicating that 41 percent of women with breast cancer thought they had brought it on themselves because of the stress in their lives.[23] The only difference from 25 years ago, and progress of a kind, is that women seem less eager to blame themselves for the stress.

Carole LeBlanc was 31 when she was diagnosed, and she has not a shadow of doubt that stress was the seedbed in which her breast lump incubated: "I am positive about that. It was a very stressful time, we lived in a basement apartment [in a city far from family], I had had a miscarriage. . . ." She desperately wanted to have another baby and was getting conflicting advice from doctors. "For me," she said, "I know it was stress. I know."[24]

Marie A. has malignant melanoma, "a ticking time bomb" that, according to her doctors, will recur. All the medical personnel she has encountered assure her that this cancer is not related to stress. She doesn't agree. She believes that the death of one of her children in

1995 so devastated her that it compromised her immune system, leaving her susceptible to disease. Her 27-year-old son was killed when he fell into a crevasse while mountain climbing, and his body was never found. "My heart will never heal," she says.[25]

The association of emotional stress to the extreme—a broken heart—and breast cancer is a theme that pervades literature. Twice in the space of a few days I encountered this connection: in a short story in *The New Yorker*, the narrator's grandmother, Agnes, dies of breast cancer. One character believes that "Agnes caught her tumors from the uranium mine on the reservation." Another thinks they came from broken ribs that never healed—"tumors take over when you don't heal right"—but the narrator says, "I wondered if my grandmother's cancer started when somebody stole her powwow regalia. Maybe the cancer started in her broken heart and then leaked out into her breasts."[26]

And Neil Peart in his memoir, *Ghost Rider: Travels on the Healing Road*, writes that when their daughter was killed in a car accident, his wife, Jackie Taylor, "[fell] to pieces and never came back together again." Within months Jackie, who was 42, was diagnosed with "terminal cancer"—"the doctors called it cancer, but, of course, it was a broken heart." She died little more than two months later.[27]

Mary Trafford speaks of a friend who she is convinced died of a broken heart that simply manifested itself in breast cancer: "Her husband died very suddenly in his late 40s, and then her son died in a boating accident at the age of 21 four years later." Two years after her son's death, the woman developed breast cancer; two years after that she was dead. "You hear this kind of story so often. I know it's all anecdotal, but you start to wonder. . . . Everyone can find stressful points in their lives, but each person deals with them in different ways, and so often breast cancer follows."[28]

Barbara McIntosh, president of a chain of china stores across Canada, says her managers, all women, most between the ages of 40 and 65, the age at which "breast cancer seems like an epidemic," chose breast cancer for the business's charity—money for breast cancer research, for treatment centres, they didn't care for what as long as it was used to help fight the disease one way or another. "They are scared to death, all of them; every single day when they wake up they think they are going to get it, so it really was a fear, at their age . . . everyone knows someone who has it.

"Women who have made it to the top [in business] have worked really, really hard to be up there and they are stressing themselves out radically." Barbara believes the same goes for women who play the social game: "Look at how much they cover up. It's a tremendous balancing act, and what suffers most is their body. . . . My mother died of breast cancer; she had a lump, she went to the doctor, the doctor said you are high-strung, it's not cancer. . . . A year later she had a mastectomy, then chemo; there was no way out. She was a cover-up artist. That was 24 years ago, and you know, I don't think the world has changed."[29]

Vladana Sistek was diagnosed with breast cancer in 2001 at the age of 39 and, like so many women, had no risk factors other than the major one—being a woman. And stress. "Stress has been part of my life for a long time," she says with understatement.[30] Born in Czechoslovakia, she escaped with her family one month after the Russian invasion. She was seven years old. She describes her adult life as one full of feelings of anger and resentment: "I'm a single parent, not had much luck with men: I was very unhappy in my first relationship, and the second one was an awful roller coaster—[he was] verbally abusive—I had to get a restraining order . . . we were together for seven years and having cancer probably is nothing compared to that relationship. I don't know how much of that immobilized my immune system."

Vladana is a psychiatric social worker and works in an acute psychiatric outpatient centre, but, she says, "I don't see the work as stressful as just juggling all the life stuff."

Although many of us accept the concept of "stress causes cancer" often without much analysis, Western scientists and researchers don't, because they need the scientific evidence, the observable connection between stress, genetic mutation and birth of a cancer cell.

But here is an interesting thing. In Traditional Chinese Medicine (TCM), stress is accepted as one of the major causes of cancer: "Emotional problems are by far the most important cause [of cancer] in Chinese Medicine. Worry, pensiveness, sadness, anger, frustration, resentment, hatred, guilt can all cause stagnation of qi [the vital energy or universal essence which flows throughout the human body and all living things] which in the long run may lead to blood stasis which forms masses."[31]

Susan Hess would agree with this. Susan was diagnosed with breast cancer three years after her husband committed suicide, leaving her to raise five young children. When she asked her doctor how long the tumour might have been growing in her breast, he told her, anywhere from three to seven years. Susan looks pensive when she talks about what might have caused it. Grief and stress sowed the seeds, she thinks. It was seven years before her diagnosis that her husband developed prostate problems, an illness that caused him to change: "The house was so full of negative energy those years," she says.[32] Then his suicide—a horrific tragedy that rocked the family off its foundations, all the more devastating because his body was discovered by one of the children. The repercussions would be grief and stress of the highest order, which snaked through the following years. Susan thinks one of the results was an immune system so damaged that the cancer grew undetected, surfacing in leering triumph to test her strength yet again, in a life already fractured with pain.

※

So here's what we do know: breast cancer is not a single- or even a double-gene disease. Unlike the genetic source of cystic fibrosis, traced by a joint team of Canadian and American scientists to a single gene on chromosome 7, breast cancer appears to be all over the genetic map. It's still classified as a genetic disease, but with serious qualifications: for those who have not inherited the breast cancer gene (a germ-line mutation), it is a *complex* genetic disease, meaning that many other factors come into play, thoroughly roiling the gene pool again. And most confounding of all, researchers now think that breast cancer is not a single disease but many, which suggests that a one-size-fits-all approach in treatments will simply not work.

A Swedish study of the incidence of 28 different cancers in 89,576 identical and fraternal twins found that environmental factors were implicated in about twice as many cancers as genetic factors. (Identical twins share the same genes while fraternal twins, on average, are just 50 percent genetically identical—the same as between siblings and between parents and offspring.) The findings suggested that even an identical twin has about a 90 percent chance of *not* getting the same cancer as his or her affected twin.[33]

"This raises the question of why aren't we doing more to identify avoidable risk factors for cancer, including occupational exposures," says Devra Lee Davis, a cancer epidemiologist at Carnegie Mellon University, Pittsburgh. "You can't choose your parents. What you can do is control your exposures in the environment."[34]

Exactly what Nicole thought. At the breast cancer conference in Kingston, she and I saw the film *Exposure: Environmental Links to Breast Cancer*, a compelling documentary on the possible connections between the environment, health and disease prevention. That same week, we heard ecologist Sandra Steingraber speak eloquently and convincingly on the growing evidence that pesticides (a term used in the literature to encompass herbicides, insecticides, fungicides and fumigants) were killing more than dandelions.

Nicole started to connect the dots: "These things are designed to kill life," she said. "They must have an effect on living tissue." On our living tissue. On us. On our children. The war on weeds, especially on the tiny battlefields of our own lawns, began to take on far more menace than an exasperating annual spring ritual.

Despite the growing body of epidemiological data implicating envi-ronmental factors in human disease, there are many who deny that the dots even belong on the same page. Weak or no science, they say. No "real" evidence of connection. These are the people who need what some call "the dead-body" proof.

In *The Silent Spring*, Rachel Carson described the fallout from an ill-conceived spraying campaign against mosquitoes in the late 1950s that wiped out all the songbirds in the area. They died in postures of grotesque convulsion, legs drawn up to their breasts, beaks gaping open around a DDT-contaminated birdbath.[35] Their tiny dead bodies provided fairly incriminating evidence of the toxicity of the chemical they'd just ingested. When the causality connection is not so direct and immediate, it is easier to refute. "However agonizing their deaths, cancer patients do not collapse around the birdbath."[36]

Patricia Hurdle remembers her father spraying DDT all around the garden and lawn where she played as a child: "The creek that we used to play in near our home suddenly, it seemed, turned a milky white and had a chemical smell to it. [A] drug company had built a plant nearby and it seems it dumped its chemicals into our play area . . . the creek. It has since been filled in."[37] Patricia has had breast cancer twice. Her sister died of it. But she can't, with any certainty, connect her cancer with the contaminants. She can only surmise.

Gerry Rogers, who made the award-winning film *My Left Breast: An Unusual Film About Breast Cancer*,[38] has similar memories. Where she grew up, the lanes behind the houses were sprayed with DDT to eradicate mosquitoes. She and her pals would run behind the trucks in the fog of pesticide, licking the sweet tasting stuff off their hands. In their small group there have been two brain tumours, several miscarriages, at least two breast cancers. Gerry, her sister and her mother all have had breast cancer. Her sister and mother both had double mastectomies; Gerry has had one breast removed. "I am the custodian of the sole breast left in this family," she says.[39]

The use of DDT reached its peak in the late 1950s and early 1960s but was banned in Canada in 1969 and in the United States three years later. What has become apparent is that banning a pesticide isn't like waving a wand and, presto, it disappears: the pesticide lingers and lingers. Thirty years later, we all have traces of it in the tissues of our bodies. The same goes for PCBs. And for atrazine, a component of many pesticides. All have been linked with cancer, but it is a controversial linkage still.

When a plant is sprayed with a common all-garden variety of herbicide such as 2,4-D (dichloro-phenoxyacetic acid), it basically grows itself to death. If you could view it in slow motion, it would be a gruesome sight: "Stems twist and contort, roots swell and leaves wither and die."[40] Cells go into warp speed growth, running amok like teenage gangs on a rampage. Sound familiar? Like cancer cells. 2,4-D is often described as cancer for plants.

For a household product, available across the counter in most garden centres and hardware stores, 2,4-D has a sinister provenance. It's not really a surprise to learn that it originated from secret research on chemical and biological weapons during the Second World War. Scientists discovered that in small doses it could be beneficial to plants, but that in large doses, it was lethal. 2,4-D was an ingredient in the infamous Agent Orange, a defoliant used in the Vietnam War which not only destroyed swaths of jungles but many of the people who lived in those jungles.

As are most pesticides and herbicides, 2,4-D is an organochlorine. A large chemical group, organochlorines are suspected of being hormone-disrupters[41]—always worrisome in relation to breast cancer—and they have other nasty attributes as well. They hang around for a long, long time, permeating the very life of our planet, and they don't stay where they are put, but drift in the air, dissolve in the water and bind to soil particles. They also accumulate in living tissue, especially fatty tissue of animals and humans, such as breasts. And one of the prices we humans pay for being at the top of the food chain is that we are at the greatest risk of accumulating high concentrations of these chemicals from all sources—not just from the air and water but from our food as well.

An exasperated toxicologist for Dow Chemical Company defends 2,4-D: "Literally hundreds of toxicology studies have given it a clean bill of health,"[42] and many defenders of pesticides say they use them all the time and don't get sick. They are looking for the immediate connection, the bang-you're-dead effect, like the lifeless birds around the birdbath. But cancers have a long latency period; they don't pop up like a cold after exposure to a germ. If they did, we'd likely have a better handle on what causes them.

The incidence of all cancers increased almost 50 percent between 1950 and 1991 in North America. Most of the upsurge has been in the last 25 years. In the decade between 1986 and 1996, breast cancer increased worldwide by 33 percent;[43] in Canada, by 25 per-cent. (The 2008 statistics indicate that incidence is still rising.) The International Agency for Research on Cancer (IARC), concludes that 80 percent of all cancers are attributable to environmental factors.[44] In its *Biennial Report 2000-2001*, it states cautiously: "Circumstantial evidence suggests that environmental exposures are breast cancer risk factors."[45]

But when does circumstantial evidence become definitive evidence? Scott Findlay, who is both a biologist and environmentalist, says that in this case, probably never. When one politician told him that we have to wait for stronger evidence before we go around banning things, his response was, "Well, you'll be waiting until hell freezes over, because you will never have stronger evidence. Just perhaps more correlation. . . ." The only way of confirming or refuting that link would be by conducting a controlled trial with human beings. Which is never going to happen.

For an increasing number of us, the proof is in the pudding, and we are the pudding. Here's where Prime Minister Jean Chrétien's definition of proof makes perfect sense: "A proof is a proof. What kind of a proof? It's a proof. A proof is a proof and when you have a good proof, it's proven."[46]

If you accept that "we are the body of evidence," as public health researcher Devra Lee Davis says, then the next step, not just for individuals but for policy makers and governments at all levels, is to adopt the precautionary principle. The precautionary principle is a major pillar of primary prevention—the stop-cancer-before-it-starts philosophy. Such strategies usually fall into two categories: the one that focuses on risk factors that might be controlled by individual action—don't smoke, don't drink alcohol, eat healthy food, exercise—and the one that focuses more on public issues such as environmental conditions, where responsibility must fall on the body politic. "Public health campaigns over the past several decades have tended to favour the former strategies focussed on an ethic of individuals taking personal responsibility for their health."[47]

But in light of the fact that one in every 100 women has been diagnosed with breast cancer over the last 15 years, it appears that such individual actions are not stemming the tide. "Are we going to get very far with exercise and diet?" Shail Verma asks, in relation to preventing breast cancer in high-risk women. "No we're not. We've done this—women are exercising more than they ever have, for heaven's sake and they're still getting breast cancer."[48]

This doesn't mean that individual acts of prevention or precaution be abandoned; it means that there are other risk factors that have to be considered as well; just as breast cancer itself can be multifocal, so can prevention strategies. A broader look at what might be controlled brings carcinogens into the picture. Some we can protect ourselves from, but from others we must look for systemic action to protect us.

But where do we start? In light of all the debate and conflicting "facts," in the face of what seems to be incontrovertible evidence, whatever the cause, that somehow we are poisoning our planet, ourselves, and worst of all, our children, where do we start? Small.

Nicole entered the fight at the community level, determined to persuade her municipality to ban cosmetic use of pesticides. She recognized that the evidence was circumstantial, but death of a dandelion was starting to look like a much more ominous murder.

"I feel overwhelmed by all there is to do to clean up this messed up world," she wrote. "I feel a sense of urgency to do it all now. I feel fearful for my three daughters, for the world I will leave in their hands. I feel guilty for having to pass it on to them in this state."[49]

She first spoke publicly about the issue to an audience of 200 people in the winter of 1998 at a ski lodge at Camp Fortune in Chelsea. Her speech galvanized the community: Action Chelsea for the Respect of the Environment/Action Chelsea pour le respect de l'environnement (ACRE) was born and persuaded the municipal council to pass a by-law, which had been languishing at the planning stage, to ban cosmetic use of pesticides. Along with a similar by-law in Hudson, Quebec—the town, coincidentally, where Nicole grew up—it was the first in Canada, showing other municipalities that it could be done. Starting small could end up launching something big. Quebec now has a province-wide ban on cosmetic use of pesticides by municipalities, and in 2008 Ontario announced similar legislation.

❧

Madeleine H. summed up the debate and all the science in a single phrase: "The genes and the mills." This is what she assumed caused her breast cancer, and her sisters', and her mother's and her aunt's. She didn't need a lab and a bunch of studies, just her own family, her own body and her own town to figure it out. The frustrating question is, Where do we go from here? Does this knowledge get us any closer to finding out what ultimately causes cancer and what might cure it?

Now, in this first decade of the 21st century, the burgeoning field of genetics holds enormous promise, even if not the clarity we at first thought. Scientists say that it is only a matter of time before we'll be able to repair individual genomes by replacing defective genes, sort of like rebuilding a car; only a matter of time before they will be able to map and solve all the mysteries of life. Maybe so, but that "matter of time" is a truly relative concept. Time in the lab is for the most part a necessary quantity stretching out like a carpet runner upon which successes and failures inch along. But for people with cancer, time is a luxury many do not have—at most, it is a tiny prayer rug upon which to kneel and pray and hope that science will find the cause and the cure of their disease before even that small comfort is whipped from under them.

We know about mutant genes; we know about proliferating cells; we know that certain genes have been identified as breast cancer genes—or maybe not. We know that it takes a series of mutations before a cell becomes cancerous. We know all these things, but we still don't know what caused our cancer. We'd stumbled into that dark room full of black cats that aren't there, and with molecular and genetic science as our flashlight, we'd established that indeed they are, but we can't actually catch them. What we do find are so many contributing factors that we are left asking ourselves, not "Why me?" not "Why not me?" but "Why not everybody?"

The issues of cause and risk factors are intertwined with all the other major issues related to breast cancer. Until we know with certainty what causes breast cancer, we cannot know with certainty how to cure it, how to control it or how to prevent it. Such an environment provides fertile ground for conflicting theories about diagnostics and early detection, about treatment protocols, about research directions and about funding priorities; it spawns disagreements about the role of the pharmaceutical industry, about the ethics of clinical trials and about the corporate role in breast cancer fundraising; it means that we must rely on the statistical guidance of epidemiology rather than on the direct medical tools of oncology to try to stem the disease; it creates an inordinate emphasis on psychosocial issues, which expand in direct correlation to the unpredictability of physical interventions; it gives rise to an explosion of information, some good, some bad, but all accessible and unfiltered by the presence of an informed interpreter; and it provides an invidious and corrosive influence to risk factors which, in lieu of confirmed cause, rule the direction of treatment research, preventative measures and lifestyle decisions of all women. Once the cause, or causes, of the disease has been truly isolated, most of these issues will vanish, or at least be focused on a clear direction with minimal debate or conflict.

3

CROSSING THE BORDER: EARLY DETECTION THROUGH SCREENING AND DIAGNOSTICS

Yendys had trouble with its spinnaker that night.
They were bringing it down in 38 knots.
Yeah, it broached, rolled on its side. These guys are pros
but they lost their bowman off the side without a life jacket.
He wasn't hooked on. He . . .
Got washed clear off the boat and then a big wave
dumped him back on the deck.
That was a lucky bugger.
That was a very lucky bugger.

—Peter Carey, *Thirty Days in Sydney*[1]

PATRICIA HURDLE'S BODY was telling her something was wrong; her doctors and her mammograms disagreed. All was well, nothing to worry about. They were wrong, she was right. She did have a tumour that technology and medical experience kept missing.

Laura G.'s lump was found in a routine screening mammogram. She had no idea anything was amiss.

45

Madeleine H. found the lumps in her breast herself, the first shortly after an all-clear doctor's examination and the second after an all-clear mammogram. Each time it was cancer.

Sharon Hampson, of the singing trio Sharon, Lois and Bram, has had breast cancer twice. And two other times, she hadn't but was told she did. She was 45, on top of the world, her life full of music and family and friends and success, when a routine mammogram rocketed her into the bleak reality of breast cancer. After a lumpectomy, she turned her back on the whole experience and got on with her life again.

Four and a half years later, another mammogram, another call from the doctor's office, another biopsy, another lumpectomy, this time followed by radiation and tamoxifen. Her treatments were piling up. Surely that would be the end of it. Maybe the end of cancer, but not the end of the crazy, frightening ride.

Six years later, an enlarged lymph node put her back on the roller coaster. The results of a core biopsy came back positive. Within three weeks she had lymph node surgery, but no cancer was found. Further investigation revealed that Sharon did not have cancer again, but another woman did, the one whose cells were biopsied the same day and analyzed in the same lab. Sharon's cells had been contaminated somehow by cancer cells from another slide. A reprieve. Of sorts.

Since Sharon is classed as high risk for the disease, she took part in a five-year study comparing MRIs to the more traditional screening procedures such as mammograms and ultrasound. In May 2003, it was déjà vu all over again, when an MRI indicated "something suspicious." There followed weeks of "yes, it's cancer . . . no, it's not . . . well, maybe it is."

"This wasn't the first time I had been called back in this study," she says.[2] But each time follow-up tests indicated that nothing was amiss. Not this time though. She had a second MRI, followed immediately by a needle biopsy. The doctor kept saying, "'It's in an awkward spot, do you mind if I take more samples?' I didn't mind—I was frozen," she says. Physically. Not emotionally.

The pathology report came back negative: all was fine. Jubilation. One day later, a second call, the "Oops call," as Sharon refers to it. "The call came on my cell phone when I was having coffee with a friend— the radiologist wasn't even sure she had hit the spot so wasn't sure she had picked up the right cells. She was strongly recommending a surgical biopsy."

Sharon turned to her own doctor (rather than doctors who were running the MRI study) to get advice in the face of all this uncertainty. "He said I had two options—a mastectomy right away, or have his people at Princess Margaret Hospital look at all the film and give a second opinion." Sharon elected to get a second opinion, which indicated that it was not cancer. Three months of fear and anxiety put to temporary rest, "temporary" being the operative word. Further tests over the next two years indicated that indeed it *was* cancer. Sharon had a mastectomy in 2005. Sometimes it's very hard to get off the roller coaster.

Women's experiences with breast cancer can be very different, though in one respect they are very much the same. It is a scary, unnerving time: the journey stutters forward in a series of stages like a train shunting and lurching from a station. You're not sure whether you will be travelling on the train, but it's the screening and diagnostic stages that have put you in the station in the first place—with a suspicious mammogram or discovery of a lump or thickening in the breast. Conflicting technology and doctors can have you getting on and off the train like a terrified yo-yo. A positive biopsy is your unwanted ticket to ride; a negative one leaves you standing in the station, thankfully waving the train on by.

The process, if not the outcome, is generally the same—the tests to confirm that there is nothing or something to worry about, and just exactly how worried to be—but of course there are exceptions to the rule. It's important to know this, because it can be disconcerting if your experience doesn't match those described in the pamphlets and handouts from the cancer clinic or your doctor's office. These are often diluted to the point of incomprehensibility in an effort not to frighten, and they describe the middle ground, the most common elements that cannot possibly include the variations and nuances of each person's experience.

Be prepared, too, to encounter debate and disagreement at every stage of the journey—from early detection through to treatment options, and indeed, even before the journey begins, with prevention and screening. You will hear the party lines, and you will hear voices of dissent, some raised in anger and frustration, others in careful questioning. The cacophony of dispute can become overwhelming, especially with so much information out there. Of course, all you want is for a single clear voice of reason to tell you the one right way to go in order to get better. But that's not how it works.

You will hear a lot about prevention. The best way to deal with breast cancer, you hear and read everywhere, is to not get it in the first place. This is one of the most persistent of admonitions, especially when it's linked with lifestyle risk factors. The prevention message isn't new—it's been around for centuries—but today it's elevated to a screaming pitch when it comes to any disease we don't know how to cure. It's puzzling why there is so much literature about it in cancer clinic waiting rooms. It is not a comfort to be reading about how you can prevent breast cancer by exercising regularly, eating properly, and having regular breast examinations when you are sitting there with a lump or thickening in your breast already; you feel as if your entire body radiates with its presence, and reading about how you could have prevented it just adds guilt to fear.

Prevention is often divided into three levels, and the ambiguity around the definition of each, particularly of primary prevention, might explain some of the confusion. According to the Surgeon General of the United States, primary prevention "generally refers to the elimination of risk factors for disease in asymptomatic persons [presenting no symptoms of disease]," secondary prevention is the early detection and treatment of disease and tertiary prevention "consists of measures to reduce impairment, disability, and suffering in people with existing disease."[3]

Cancer Care Ontario's Prevention Blueprint (2000) is more precise: "cancer prevention includes two main strategies:

- "eliminating the causes of cancer and preventing the disease from getting started in the first place and
- screening to find cancer and its precursors so that it can be treated easily and effectively."[4]

The yoking of prevention and early detection—have an annual screening mammogram or practise breast self-examination to prevent cancer—is an odd coupling since, of course, once a cancer is detected, it can't be prevented. It's the old slamming the barn door after the horse has bolted routine. "Early detection is the best prevention" is a catchy slogan, but it doesn't stand up to scrutiny. What it is trying to convey is the theory that you can get a jump on the disease, with better odds for success, the earlier the cancer is discovered. But, however you define it, this is not prevention.

ꙮ

Generally, experts believe that there is a much better prognosis for women whose cancer is detected early, when the tumour is still small and perhaps the cancer cells have not left the primary site and invaded the lymph system or other organs. The qualifier "generally" is important, because in some cases the size of the tumour doesn't matter; it's the aggressiveness of the cancer that does, and, even if detected early, it may be already too late to contain it. (That is, if it were going to go anywhere at all. Researchers think that some cancers might never plan to colonize, content to sit forever where they first appear.) It is a conundrum not only for women but for doctors trying to advise them on treatment. Do you opt for aggressive treatment even when the cancer is found early and the tumour is contained and tiny? Or do you wait and see, hoping that it will never develop into anything even remotely life-threatening? Science can't give us one clear direction yet; it can and does give us lots of directions to choose from, though.

Here's where you'll encounter the first rumblings of disagreement. The emphasis on the need to find a tumour early emerged in the opening decades of the 20th century, when the stigma of the disease kept many women silent about the cancer ulcerating their breasts, preferring to go to the grave than to a doctor. Their tumours could be the size of oranges before they might be persuaded to go for treatment, and by then, for most, it was way too late. Through the next few decades, detection relied on visual observation and touch, not a particularly early warning system. Mammography, introduced in the 1960s, was the tool that was going to make early detection viable.

The importance of early detection is still under question though; advances in the understanding of the biology of cancer indicate that once a breast tumour is big enough to be detectable, the cancer has already been there for six to eight or ten years. Maybe even longer. A 30-year study in the United States established that the median doubling time of a tumour was 260 days. The actual range though was huge: the fastest tumour doubled in 10 days, the slowest in 7,051 days—almost 20 years.[5] The implications of these figures reach farther than the importance of, or lack of, early detection—they reach into the entire world of treatment, going far to explain why the successes and failures of various therapies are so unpredictable. Take a woman who has a tumour that doubles every 30 days. Twenty-three cell generations later, the tumour might be visible on a mammogram but by then will contain billions of cancer cells. The question is, are tumours any more likely to metastasize after 23 doublings than, say, after 12? Early detection rests on the assumption that they are.

Early detection also assumes that the smaller the lump, the less serious it is. Not necessarily so: small tumours can be extremely aggressive, and large ones can be less so; some large masses can include tissue that the body forms to protect itself against the cancer.[6]

No matter, say some: if the tumour can be removed, and any errant cancer cells mopped up with adjuvant therapy (chemotherapy, radiation and/or hormone therapy), it is still possible to prevent metastasis— cancer spread to the bones or vital organs. And the countervailing theory to *that* is the belief held by some microbiologists that as soon as cancer cells begin their immortal, insanely replicating journey, they immediately have the wherewithal to metastasize—the murderous ability to permeate the walls of other cells, escape into the blood and lymph systems and move on out to colonize vital organs.

Whatever the biology, early detection is the mantra of public awareness campaigns, which include in their literature some pretty convincing, if very general, statistics: the five-year survival rate decreases from 95 percent for cancers treated at an early stage to 36 percent for cancers that have spread to surrounding tissue and to 7 percent for late-stage cancers that have spread to distant organs.[7]

SCREENING

Screening is "the process of looking at healthy people with no symptoms in order to pick up early signs of disease."[8] This is known as "primary prevention"; some call it trawling. It is a three-pronged approach: breast self-examination, regular physical examinations by doctors and mammography. You will hear arguments about the effectiveness, reliability and usefulness of all three.

Breast Self-Examination (BSE)

Breast self-examinations have been recommended for years as the obvious first step in early detection. What at first blush appears to be common-sensical advice was knocked on its ear by the findings of two large studies conducted in the 1990s. The first tracked 267,040 female factory workers in China, half of whom were taught how to examine their breasts for lumps, thickening or puckering that might indicate a problem, the other half not. After five years, approximately equal numbers of breast cancer were detected in each group, the cancers found in the BSE group were not discovered earlier than in the control group and the death rates for each group were exactly equal. Results of a similar study carried out in Russia also showed no advantage to breast self-examination.

In September 2002, the Canadian Task Force on Preventive Health Care analyzed the findings of these and various other studies concluded that BSE was worse than ineffective. For example, in the Chinese study, the BSE group found more lumps than the other group (1,457 versus 623), but 90 percent of these lumps were benign, thus considerably stressing their owners with unnecessary biopsies and worry. The Task Force recommendation was clear, if wordy: "Because there is fair evidence of no benefit, and good evidence of harm, there is fair evidence to recommend that routine teaching of BSE be excluded from the periodic health examination of women" in all age groups. It added a rather peculiar corollary though: "*Important note:* Although the evidence indicates no benefit from routine instruction, some women will ask to be taught BSE. The potential benefits and harms should be discussed with the woman, and if BSE is taught, care must be taken to ensure she performs BSE in a proficient manner."[9]

The Task Force's study authors were roundly criticized because they offered no replacement for BSE and because "the results of the study really left women dangling," says Laurie Beitel, president of Breast Cancer Action in Saskatchewan. "For years we've been saying that we know our bodies best and so, if there's something unusual, we're the ones who will pick it up, so we should be doing [BSE] monthly."[10]

In response to the controversy stirred up by the Chinese and Russian studies and subsequent analyses, the Canadian Breast Cancer Foundation and the Canadian Cancer Society issued position statements supporting BSE. But the debate continues (see introduction).

Patricia Hurdle knows her own body. "I just didn't listen to it," she says ruefully.[11] She was diagnosed with breast cancer four months after her sister died of it. Patricia had kept a diary for years, as a yoga practice, to record dreams, fears, thoughts and daily happenings as a way of getting to meditation. She went back to her journals of five years before, written when her sister had been diagnosed. She found something she had forgotten about: "I had written 'I feel something in my left armpit, something is pulling in my left breast, oh my god, is there something?'"

Perhaps it was just her imagination, overreaction because of her sister's situation. A mammogram indicated that nothing was there. "I said to myself, 'Oh, it's all in my mind, I'm just paranoid.'" Another year passed and during that time her diaries showed that she'd dream about cancer over and over. She kept feeling a pulling sensation in her breast, and then a thickening. "I went back each year [for a mammogram and check-up], because of my family history, and they'd say, it's nothing. No, it looks fine, [the] mammogram is fine. Technology and the doctors all said there is nothing there, but I was recording in my diary, my body was clearly telling me there was, but I didn't want to hear it, so I believed them."

In June 1998, Patricia went for her annual check-up. This time, technology had finally caught up: the mammogram detected the tumour she had felt all along.

Some forms of breast cancer, however, are undetectable in a self-examination. You are unlikely to find a ductal carcinoma in situ (DCIS) because it usually doesn't form a lump. (DCIS is cancer cells that have grown in the duct but not beyond their site of origin; it is sometimes called precancer.) Same with lobular carcinoma in situ (LCIS)—abnormal cells within the lobule that don't form lumps but can serve as a marker for possible future cancer. These might show up on a mammogram as a cluster of tiny little dots, like a scatter of salt.

Inflammatory breast cancer is normally undetectable through BSE because it forms in nests or sheets rather than in solid tumours. It is often misdiagnosed as mastitis (inflammation of the breast) because some of its symptoms are similar: a rapid swelling of the whole breast;

thickening breast tissue; redness, blotchiness or a rash; and persistent itching of the breast or nipple. Other signs can include pain, heat, dimpling or ridging of the breast, flattening or retracting of the nipple, nipple discharge or change of the pigmented area of the nipple. These symptoms are not what we are usually taught to look for in examining our breasts for cancer. (A simple skin biopsy will confirm whether they are symptomatic of a benign condition or something more sinister.)

Moncton's Madeleine H. has had breast cancer twice. She had a mastectomy eight years ago; the cancer came back at the site of the incision seven years later. "You know, they say now that self-examination is no good? Well I found both lumps myself. And I'd just been to the doctor the week before and he examined me and he didn't find anything. Even the first mammogram for the first lump came back "normal breast tissue," but I could feel the lump, and it was a good size, so I don't have too much faith in mammograms. It didn't show up the second time either, but there wasn't enough flesh for the poor [technician] to get hold of—there's just skin and bone there now."[12]

Marcia Frank was even more outspoken. Breast cancer had been a spectre in her life from an early age. Her mother had died of it, and she'd been on the watch for it ever since. She was vigilant, she said, did everything the books say. "Early detection? Oh, puhleese. Don't talk to me about early detection. I've been mammographied, palpated and poked nearly to death over the last five years, and this lump did not show up. I kept going back, saying I think there is something wrong, it hurts, it feels funny. When the nipple inverted and the breast started puckering, they said that a biopsy was needed."[13] She had surgery and 27 lymph nodes removed. All were cancerous. The disease was already racing through her body.

The controversy stirred up about BSE is the unfortunate result of the fine-tuned tools of science being thrust into an area where they can't work, for the fundamental reason that "science cannot comprehend what it cannot measure."[14] The lack of controls of the many variables in these studies—the very unruliness of human nature—make the results suspect. And when they are taken as reason for encouraging women to abandon the commonsense practice of checking their own breasts for changes, they are more than suspect: they are harmful.

Breast Examination by a Doctor

If your doctor knows how to do a breast examination properly, it is a good screening method, especially in combination with a mammogram. The problem is that most doctors, except for breast surgeons, have not been trained to do thorough physical breast exams. And an incomplete examination is worse than none at all because of the false assurances it can elicit, possibly delaying the finding of a lump, as happened with Marcia and Patricia. I once was examined by a young resident at a big teaching hospital in Ottawa. He seemed terrified to touch me, standing as far away as he could while still making contact. His arms were so long, it became a surreal version of distance learning. I kept telling him it was okay, but his flaming cheeks and averted eyes indicated that he was not reassured. He didn't find a lump; he could barely find me.

Mammography

Mammography is an X-ray that produces pictures of the soft tissue within the breast. Screening mammography is a medical fixture now; national screening programs are supported by governments in most Western countries. In Canada, organized breast screening programs, which began rolling out across the country in 1986, are now nationwide. All offer screening for women from the ages of 50 to 69 and some will screen women from the ages of 40 to 74. A study of the data from screening programs in Canada in 1997–1998 showed that of 529,875 women aged 50 to 69, "on average, 6.7 and 4.2 cancers were found per 1,000 screens in the first and subsequent screening rounds, respectively."[15]

No other early detection technique has been quite so mired in controversy, both about its efficacy and its safety, as routine screening mammography. One doctor calls it "the worst idea medicine ever had . . . the assumption is that picking cancer up early is a good thing, but in many cases it would have shown itself anyway—all screening does is let a woman know she has cancer for longer."[16] At the other extreme, proponents of screening mammography claim it saves thousands of lives. (There is often confusion about mammography because it plays two roles—as a screening tool for healthy women, which is the focus of most of the fuss, and as a diagnostic tool for women who already have "something suspicious.") The various arguments have polarized with each passing study, beleaguering women already dealing with a passel of other issues and decisions. Here's how it goes:

Routine screening mammograms:
- save lives by detecting breast cancers early;
- are a waste of public money and are virtually useless because they produce too many false positive results and miss as many real problems;
- actually cause cancer through exposure to radiation;
- are a conspiracy, foisted on the public by the medical establishment or by the greedy corporations that produce the machines and the film;
- are useless in detecting cancer in premenopausal women ("officially" those under the age of 50) but are useful in detecting cancers in post-menopausal women;
- are useful for detecting early cancers in women between ages 40 and 50; and
- detect precancers or early cancer conditions that might never have developed into invasive tumours.

Each side has studies to support its claims. Each year there are new studies, contradicting earlier ones.

Dr. Susan Love, an American breast surgeon and one of the most reliable, intelligent and credible players in the world of breast cancer today, says, "There is no argument that every woman over 50 should be having yearly mammography."[17] I was startled to read this until I realized that she was stating her opinion—that there *should* be no argument. But indeed there is. In 1995, Canadian researchers C.J. Wright and C.B. Mueller published the results of their analysis of breast cancer screening studies to date, showing that mammography does not save lives and subjects women to the unnecessary stress and anxiety of further tests because of so many false positives.[18] Some research suggests that 85 percent of initial "abnormal" findings in the Canadian screening programs are fine on callback.[19] That's a lot of stress and anxiety.

Wright and Mueller were unequivocal in their recommendation: "Since the benefit achieved is marginal, the harm caused is substantial, and the costs incurred are enormous, we suggest that public funding for breast cancer screening in any age group is not justifiable." In case anyone misunderstood their message, they elaborated: women have "been duped by the medical community overselling the benefits of the tool because it had nothing else to offer."[20] Critics of the study were savage, claiming that it was statistically naïve and riddled with inaccuracies.

John William Gofman, chair of the Committee for Nuclear Responsibility in the United States, a doctor and professor emeritus of molecular and cell biology at the University of California, has been making the same argument for years, not because he believes mammograms are useless as a screening tool but because he believes they actually cause more cancer than they detect due to repeated exposure to radiation.[21] Although the radiation dosages have greatly decreased over the years, they still represent a considerable risk. Rosalie Bertell, anti–nuclear energy and radiation activist and founder of several international medical commissions, says the radiation dosages are far higher than "considerable." At the First World Conference on Breast Cancer in Kingston, she told a spellbound audience that a four-film mammogram exposes the breast to 1,000 times more radiation than a chest X-ray, and that breast tissue is particularly vulnerable to radiation damage that can break down the DNA causing mutations in genetic material.

In January 2000, a meta-analysis of all existing clinical trials of mammography, entitled "Is screening for breast cancer with mammography justifiable?" shook the breast cancer world anew, supporting the findings of the Canadian researchers Wright and Mueller. The study authors, Dr. Peter Gøetzsche and Ole Olsen of the Nordic Cochrane Collaboration in Copenhagen, conclude that "there is no reliable evidence that screening decreases breast-cancer mortality."[22]

The response from critics was immediate. "Breast cancer screening is worthwhile," wrote Stephen W. Duffy, MRC Biostatistics Unit, Institute of Public Health, Cambridge, England. "Ill-considered publications must not be allowed to cause anxiety to women invited to screening, nor to damage the morale of the staff who provide the screening. People need to know that Gøetzsche and Olsen's paper is not worth a moment's attention."[23] So the authors revisited their research and confirmed their findings a year later, flying directly into the face of the medical establishment in 22 countries married to screening mammography.[24] The *New York Times* weighed in with an editorial questioning whether we'd ever get the goods on mammography: "It may not be easy to get a truly independent review. Mammography has been so strongly endorsed by the cancer establishment and has become a significant source of revenue and patients for many hospitals and doctors that it might be difficult to excise without overwhelming evidence that it is dangerous."[25]

This really rattled some cages. Four days later, 10 US groups, including the American Cancer Society and the American Medical Association, took out a full-page advertisement in the *Times* supporting mammography. It was beginning to look like a schoolyard brawl, not over marbles but over women's lives.

Experts now say that women have to decide for themselves whether to have screening mammograms. It's not surprising that many are perplexed by this lack of direction from experts who for the last 25 years had been certain that screening mammography was the best way to catch breast cancer early. "It is as if a group of trusting passengers boarded a ferry that advertised a quick and safe passage to the opposite shore, but mid-voyage, a thick fog developed, the radar failed, and the crew started to fight over the proper direction. And so the captain announced that the passengers would now have to decide for themselves on the proper course forward."[26]

Assuming that early detection is a good thing and that mammography is safe, the next question is, at what age should you have one? The answer depends on who you ask. The reason the question even comes up is this: there seems to be *some* agreement among *some* health practitioners that, at least for women in the 50-to-69-year age group, regular screening mammograms do help reduce breast cancer deaths by about one-third. Although this statistic is contested as well, it is the number you will find most often in the literature. In March 2002, WHO's International Agency for Research on Cancer analyzed the various mammography studies and, contrary to the Nordic Cochrane Collaboration's findings, found sufficient evidence that the death rates for women in this age group can be reduced by 35 percent if they have regular mammograms. One of the most disturbing aspects of all this brouhaha is that the conflicting findings rise out of the same data: the WHO group took "a fresh look at old studies."[27] In other words, the numbers don't change but the interpretations do, a situation familiar to scientists but bewildering to patients.

The data get even murkier when it comes to the efficacy of screening mammography for women under 50. It may be that the denser breast tissue of premenopausal women masks cancer, which often shows up as dense areas in an X-ray. After menopause, the tissue becomes fatty and tumours are easier to detect. This isn't true in all cases though, and mammograms *can* detect tumours in younger women. The proponents of early mammography say that since cancers that occur in premenopausal women are usually more virulent and faster growing than those found in post-menopausal women, it is crucial to find them early. The critics point out that more than one-fourth of invasive breast cancers in the younger age group are not detected by mammography, a dangerous situation because a false negative mammogram could delay diagnosis or treatment.[28]

In 1997, the US National Cancer Institute (NCI) convened a conference of experts to decide whether the recommended screening guidelines should be expanded to include women in their 40s. "After extensive research, presentations, and debate the consensus was that there was not enough evidence to recommend universal screening and that each woman would need to decide for herself—with the help of her doctor—whether to be screened."[29] Well, that put the cat among the pigeons. Proponents of mammography were furious—one even termed this conclusion a death sentence for women younger than 50.[30] Many were highly critical of the lack of direction being provided to women wondering what to do, whom to believe. Others, Dr. Love included, commended the experts for their honesty in how they dealt with the issue of screening mammography as a public policy issue, while recognizing that it doesn't solve the problem for individual women.

In September 2002, a group of Canadian investigators, led by Anthony Miller, professor emeritus at the University of Toronto, continued the investigation and concluded that annual mammograms for women between the ages of 40 and 49 did not help reduce deaths from breast cancer. The Canadian National Breast Screening Study looked at 50,000 women at 15 clinic sites. The study results created an uproar—again—with breast cancer organizations scrambling to come up with a position on the issue. The dispute was highlighted by the publication of a report by the United States Preventive Services Task Force, which concluded that annual screening mammograms for women in their 40s *were* of benefit. This study, which combined results of eight randomized controlled trials of screening mammograms worldwide, involving half a million women, stated that a woman who starts having mammograms in her 40s "is about 15% less likely to die of breast cancer."[31]

These two studies hit the airwaves in the same week. The media had a field day reporting the outrage of supporters and critics of both studies, who busily savaged each other in the press.

While some breast cancer organizations (including the NCI) wobbled on their official stances, the Canadian Breast Cancer Network quickly issued a press release unequivocally supporting routine mammograms for Canadian women aged 40 and older. Nevertheless, "most medical organizations now discourage screening premenopausal women under 50, except for those designated 'high risk.' Despite repeated failures of studies to show a benefit, however, a few influential groups in the medical community still promote breast screening from age 40 onwards. As a result, two contradictory sets of official guidelines for mammography screening are now in circulation."[32] The debate goes on.

These disagreements are unsettling, both for women trying to stay healthy and out of the breast cancer world, and for doctors who are trying to help them. They affect organizations mandated to set public policy and cause angst among groups trying to provide leadership in the breast cancer community. But they become mere statistical skirmishes between researchers compared with the most troubling controversy about screening mammography—that of overdetection—the finding of "cancers" so early that might never become cancer at all. Here, women are directly affected, not just by the pinpricks of unease about the efficacy and safety of mammograms for women of any age but by the deep and real wounds resulting from overzealous early detection.

First are the scares: countless times women are called back after a "suspicious" mammogram, or are told to wait in the changing cubicle with the ambiguous instruction from the technician, "Don't get dressed until I make sure these X-rays are okay." What she usually means is that she needs to check that the image is in focus, that you didn't move just as she took the X-ray and that the machine was operating correctly. But she could also have spotted something suspicious, not *with* the film, but *on* the film, and so is having another look to decide whether to do a second set of X-rays for the radiologist. This is scary stuff. Most of the time, she comes back with a cheery, "Okay, you can get dressed now. Off you go." But sometimes, she will take more X-rays without ever really explaining why.

Elodie d'Ombrain had been going to the Ville Marie Multi-disciplinary Breast Center in Montreal for years for her annual mammo-gram and check-up. All clear each time. We all do it, even women who have never had breast cancer, who aren't even at high risk for the disease, but who have taken the "early detection is prevention" message to heart. We fit our annual check-ups in between the various other items of a daily routine: before a work presentation, after a dentist appointment, before a parent-teacher interview, after lunch with a friend. And usually that's where it stays, another unremarkable item on our to-do list. Until the time the technician doesn't say, "Off you go, see you next year."

Elodie's agenda for the day was knocked endways when she was called into the radiologist's office at the clinic soon after her mammo-gram and told that there was something suspicious—tiny white dots, probably calcification, something to watch. Could it be cancer? Well, yes, but unlikely. Let's watch it for six months.

We are counselled not to worry in such circumstances: "Don't be alarmed if your physician recommends waiting six months and taking a second mammogram. This is a reasonable time to show changes in an ambiguous reading and calcifications, even if cancerous, are not likely to pose immediate danger."[33] The thing is, we do worry, we are alarmed. Hard not to be. Elodie consulted with another physician in her hometown, who gave the same advice, so she settled down not to worry for six months.

In July she went back for the follow-up mammogram, which confirmed that the white dots were noncancerous calcifications and that all was okay. But six months is a long time to have the spectre of breast cancer hovering, no matter how far back in your subconscious. Elodie went to the Ritz Carlton hotel and treated herself to champagne and fois gras in celebration of the lifting of the cloud she had convinced herself was not even on her radar. I can't imagine a woman who wouldn't worry, at least in the pre-dawn hours, when told that something was up with her mammogram. That worry though is perhaps a small price to pay for early warning of a real problem.

For many women, the six-month follow-up mammogram confirms something more sinister: with screening mammography this is, increasingly, the detection of ductal carcinoma in situ (DCIS) or lobular carcinoma in situ (LCIS). DCIS and LCIS are the new kids on the block, ushered into the limelight by improved screening mammograms. In Canada, DCIS now accounts for between 20 and 25 percent of breast cancer diagnoses. But many experts believe these cases are not yet breast cancer, and may never become so. Susan Love calls these conditions "precancers," a preferred nomenclature that has brought her into conflict with many of her colleagues who believe in calling a spade a spade, whether it's going to dig a grave or not. Not only do doctors disagree on what to call these conditions, they disagree on how to treat them.

"As few as one in four women with DCIS may go on to develop an invasive tumour, yet a DCIS diagnosis is one of the most common reasons a woman undergoes a mastectomy."[34] The average size of tumours picked up by mammography has steadily decreased over the last 20 years as the technology has improved. Some of these would never have become symptomatic, or might have disappeared on their own. But even as mammography detects tinier and tinier lumps— some the size of pencil dots—many doctors feel they have no choice but to treat them, and to do so as if they all are potentially fatal.

In 2001, standard treatment recommendations for DCIS were added to the Canadian Clinical Practice Guidelines for breast cancer: mastectomy or, the preferred option, lumpectomy followed by radiation. These are highly invasive procedures for a condition that might not develop in the first place. It is a tough call, and at the moment there are no answers, just questions—another example of technology in one area outstripping knowledge in another. For every woman saved through early diagnosis, many others receive painful, disfiguring and potentially dangerous treatments for something that poses little or no threat: "tumours that they might die with, not of."[35]

Professor Baum, a British breast cancer surgeon, sums up the dilemma well: "The best estimate is that you will need to screen 1,000 women over 50 for 10 years to save one life. The value of one life saved is infinite; you can't put a price on it. But hundreds of women will suffer false alarms, unnecessary surgery and over-treatment as a result of screening. Women should be treated as intelligent human beings, not coerced into screening."[36] In other words, it's your decision.

In the meantime, announcements of pending new screening methods appear regularly, but most are a long way off from regular use.[37] Until one of these new methods pans out, mammography is the best screening technique we've got. For some, that's beside the point. "It seems odd that we go trawling our healthy population," says one activist. "Why go looking for a disease? Why not use the money and expertise that we have to deal with women who have symptoms?"[38] Exactly what some scientists and researchers, bone-weary of the debate, are asking.

In March 2002, two leading researchers in the Canadian breast cancer world pleaded for an end to the fighting: "It is time for the angst about breast cancer to move from screening to questions of molecular diagnoses, aetiology, selection of optimum therapy, and improved survival for women in a more timely and cost-effective way."[39] Sounds like a plan.

DIAGNOSTICS

If something suspicious has been found during screening, diagnostics is the next stage in the breast cancer journey. It is a stage that can have you stumbling with fear or leaping with relief, depending on the outcome. It includes mammography again, as well as other imaging tools, and biopsies, which are the passports into the new world. You might be sent for an ultrasound or an MRI (magnetic resonance imaging) scan, which has been around for a couple of decades but is being used more and more as a tool in breast cancer diagnoses. There is still debate about its usefulness in screening because of the number of false positives it produces.

MRI Scanning

During an MRI for breast cancer, you lie on your stomach inside a scanner, encompassed by a body-sized magnet that detects the electro-magnetic qualities of the body's cells and then sends this information to a computer, which produces an image. Before the procedure, you are injected with a dye as a contrast agent to highlight breast abnormalities. As the dye travels throughout your body, it is picked up most quickly by cancerous tumours, since they have more blood vessels than normal tissue. These tumours show up as bright spots on the MRI scan.

An MRI scan is a very noisy affair; you are given heavy ear protectors to wear, but the banging still penetrates as if someone were knocking wildly at the door. You'll hear a series of short bursts of noise at first as the technician customizes the machine to your body, more specifically, to your hydrogen molecules. Then the noise settles to long bursts, all the while a rumble in the background, which sounds like a clothes dryer with a running shoe thumping around in it.

The procedure usually lasts about 30 minutes to an hour, depend-ing on the hospital or centre. Some will do both breasts at the same time, if that is required; others do one at a time, on different days, because your body must be clear of the dye before the second proce-dure can be done.

I had an MRI, not a breast cancer scan but one to see if there was anything "untoward" going on in my right ear, and was startled when the technician fitted a kind of cage over my head, a bit like Hannibal Lecter's mask but without the teeth. The technician explained that this was the antennae, not something to keep me from biting anyone. (An antennae is not used in a breast cancer MRI.) The whole procedure is completely painless but could be a bit of an ordeal if you are claustrophobic. You are advised to keep your eyes shut if you think the enclosed space is going to get to you, which of course means that your eyes will immediately spring wide open. However, you do have a panic button to push if it gets to be too much, and the technicians will haul you out immediately.

CT Scanning

CT (computerized tomography) scanning, also called CAT (computerized axial tomography) scanning, uses X-rays and a computer to produce detailed cross-sectional images. This procedure is used not so much for first-line investigation of breast tumours as it is to check, after a confirmed diagnosis, for metastasis elsewhere.

Blood Tests

Blood tests for breast cancer are no longer often used for women with primary breast cancer because they are not specific or sensitive enough to be reliable in detecting microscopic metastases. "Too many false positives and false negatives," my GP said, dismissing the blood tests that I had relied on for years after treatment for primary breast cancer and that confirmed each time, "Yes, we have no cancer today." When my doctor stopped the test, it was as if she'd taken away an old friend who had reassured me every six months that so far I was free of recurrence.

Blood tests are, however, useful for women with metastatic disease, because the markers in the blood tend to go up when metastasis is extensive. In these cases, blood tests can be used as a basis to make adjustments to treatment.

Thermography

Thermography (infrared imaging) is gaining popularity again after being sidelined years ago by mammography proponents. Newer, more reliable machines have helped overcome resistance to this method, which measures heat in the form of infrared radiation coming off the body, detecting cancer cells at an early stage of reproduction, when they begin to create their own blood supply. The more blood circulation, the more heat shows up in the thermogram. Unlike mammography, infrared imaging does not require radiation, compression, contact or intravenous access—all pluses. However, in some quarters, critics still claim it is not as accurate as mammography.

PET Scanning

PET (positron emission tomography) scanning is also attracting attention. This technique uses radiation to detect glucose-filled tumours. All tissues need glucose to survive, but cancer cells need more than normal cells because of their rapid development. The theory is that since cancer cells are faster growing and use more glucose, they will show up better on the scan. Because the PET scanners are so expensive, they are still available only in large cancer centres. Also, there is discussion about whether the procedure is any better than mammography.

Ductal Lavage

Ductal lavage is a relatively new diagnostic method in which fluid is drawn from the milk ducts in the breast by suction through a catheter inserted into the nipple, and then examined for cancer cells. Sounds gruesome, but women in clinical trials of this procedure claim it is only moderately uncomfortable.

❧

Depending on the cancer centre, these various diagnostic tests are used for screening in women at high risk for cancer, though more often they are used after initial screening has located a potential problem. Like hide and seek, the doctors know that there is something lurking in your breast; now they have to pinpoint it, assess whether it's benign or malignant, and if malignant, how big it is and whether it is likely to come roaring out of its lair to settle in other parts of your body. What you are hoping for at this stage—hoping and praying and bargaining for with God or Allah or Buddha or maybe even your good luck jade toad—is that you will get home free.

You or your doctor or a screening device has detected something suspicious; usually it's a lump. If it is round and smooth, it's probably a cyst, which has fluid in it rather than consisting of solid mass, or it's a fibroadenoma, a benign fibrous tumour most common in young women. An ultrasound will confirm which of these two it is. If a mammogram shows the lump to have jagged, distinct radiating strands pulling inward, it's likely to be cancer. That's what the books say. And most of the time, they are right. But there are those of us who can't seem to go by the book. The lump I had was nearly certainly a cyst, the surgeon told me. "Nearly certainly" in medical lingo means "99 percent sure." What it often means is that someone is fully in the grip of wishful thinking. The lump didn't show up on the mammogram, even though I could feel it (an explanation offered later for this was that the lump was too high to get caught in the vice that squished my breast flat for the camera), so there was no certainty that it had smooth edges. It felt smooth. It felt like a large, wobbly pea. None of the books I consulted explained what a pea-shaped lump might mean; I did learn later that the wobbliness was probably a good thing, meaning that the lump wasn't embedded in the muscle. It is not a good sign if the lump is fixed, if it doesn't move when palpated. Turned out "wobbly" wasn't either. It was cancer.

Nancy Lee didn't go by the book either. A tiny lump in her breast sent her to the doctor. It was about the size of a peppercorn but definitely a lump. Probably nothing to worry about, she was told. It *was* something to worry about: it was DCIS, which was surprising, since the usual presentation of such an early condition is not a lump at all but abnormalities no bigger than a pencil tip. A biopsy confirmed the diagnosis, and she had a lumpectomy followed by radiation treatments. This was a tough experience, no question, but not quite so nasty as that of a woman in Britain who was told she should have a full mastectomy, after a routine screening mammogram found clusters of DCIS in her breast. "They didn't offer me any options: just that the whole breast should come off. Somewhere in there, they said that not all DCIS becomes full-blown cancer but that they treat it as if it would." The woman was devastated and went for a second opinion to another oncologist, a doctor who obviously had some work to do on her people skills. "I don't know why you've come to see me," she said. "We can't tell you what you've got until it's off and in the pot."[40]

Biopsies aren't usually described as the cutting off of a part of you and putting it in a pot to see what's there. But they are procedures in which bits or all of the lump are removed and sent to a pathologist for examination. Currently there are four types of biopsy with some variations within each category. A needle biopsy takes a few cells out of the lump (a fine needle aspiration [FNA] may be used to extract fluid, if there is any); a core biopsy, done with a larger needle and guided either by ultrasound or X-ray, cuts out a bigger chunk of tissue; an incisional biopsy carves out a bigger piece yet and the excisional biopsy takes out the whole lump. (This last is sometimes confused with a "lumpectomy," the surgical procedure to remove a confirmed malignant tumour and surrounding margins. A lumpectomy is not a diagnostic procedure but part of a treatment protocol.)

I had a needle biopsy. The books say, "The surgeon will anaesthetize the breast with a small amount of lidocaine and then use a needle and syringe to try to get a few cells."[41] My surgeon must not have read those books. No anaesthetic. He tried to draw fluid off the lump, with no luck, suggesting that it might not be a cyst after all. When the cells he did manage to collect were sent to the pathology lab for examination, the results came back negative: no cancer. Three months later, when my intuitive and watchful GP sent me to the breast surgeon for a second biopsy, the results came back positive. Cancer. How could this be? A fine needle aspiration removes only a few cells and so can miss cancerous ones. Biopsies are almost but not completely failsafe; the most reliable are core biopsies and more extensive surgical biopsies because they give more to the pathologist to examine.

A positive biopsy feels as if you've been washed right off the deck of your old life without a life jacket. Even as you flounder in the sea, it is impossible not to harbour the hope that there has been a mistake, that your doctor will phone and say that the lab mixed up the slides, that the pathologist has had a closer look and all is fine, or that surgery will find no cancer. There isn't one of us who wouldn't think there was a tiny chance that, like the sailor in the Hobart Yacht Race who was swept out to sea and then dumped right back into the boat, we could be given our old life back. Even though biopsies are rarely wrong in the right way—a positive one turning out to be negative when the full lump has been removed and examined—that doesn't stop you from wishing, hoping and praying that it will be. And it does happen.

Laura G. harboured such hopes, undergoing a lumpectomy with high expectations—the champagne was already chilling in the fridge—that the lump would be benign despite the biopsy evidence eight months before.

Laura had pinned her hopes on a friend's experience, a woman who *was* washed back onto her boat. Her friend told her, "I went through this two years ago. I had a biopsy and they told me I had cancer. Nine months of hell—I finally had a lumpectomy, but I didn't have the nodes removed, and the pathology of the lump indicated no cancer." Her doctor said that this was not the first time such a misdiagnosis had happened.

Hoping, wishing, praying—nothing wrong with any of these. Hope is good. Wishing and praying are good. But hope is crucial. Hope is the main man. Remember that there *are* exceptions to the rules all the time. Never discount the slim possibilities, because they happen. Some would say that faced with such odds, this would be false hope. Not necessarily.

I remember asking my surgeon if there was any chance that the second biopsy, which had come back positive, could be wrong, and that when he took out the lump it might be benign. He frowned, his eyes slid away from mine, he fiddled with a pencil, all in an attempt to let me down easily. Very unlikely, he said. He was 99 percent certain that he would find malignancy, just as the biopsy indicated. But I was hanging on to that other "99 percent certain" of his that had been 100 percent wrong, when he'd told me that the second biopsy would almost certainly come back negative and it came back positive. So couldn't it happen again, only this time the flipside—that the 99 percent certain would give way to the possible 1 percent? It didn't, but oddly, my hope was not shaken so much as redirected: I carried it, or the second generation of it, with me to the next stage, when I waited for the results of the lymph node excision. Once again, what I hoped for didn't happen. Two nodes had cancer cells in them. So I moved into third generation hope—that I'd survive first, the treatment, second, the cancer. And my hope, for all sorts of reasons, strengthened at each stage. Maybe it was all the practice.

Was this was misplaced hope, false hope? Who can say. That's the thing about hope: you can only label it after the fact. Until then, it carries you like a lifebuoy, which is a whole lot better than drowning. This may seem like nothing more than mind games. Perhaps. But if mind games help, then what's wrong with playing them?

4 TREATMENTS OF DIRECT ASSAULT: THE REIGNING TRIUMVIRATE

*Most of the traits and skills you bring with you from your native life
are irrelevant, while strange new attributes suddenly matter.
Beautiful hair is irrelevant. Permanent veins along the soft skin
at the fold of your arm are highly prized. The ability to cook
a delicious meal in thirty minutes is irrelevant. The ability to lie
completely motionless on a hard platform for half an hour while
your bones are scanned for signs of tumor is, conversely, quite useful.*

—Sandra Steingraber, *Living Downstream*[1]

WHEN NICOLE'S DIAGNOSIS WAS CONFIRMED, she already knew
the established route. She saw breast cancer patients all the time in her
medical practice, and she was well acquainted with this wretched
disease, but from the other side, the outside. She knew the research,
the stats, the prognoses, the current clinical trials. She saw daily the
pain and fear caused by diagnoses, the confusion of treatment options,
the disfigurement of surgery, the nausea of chemotherapy and the
burns and depression of radiation. It was a shock to have to apply this

knowledge and experience to herself, but she did not hesitate. Within hours of confirmation of the malignancy she embarked on one of the first established stages of the treatment trail—a full mastectomy.

Nancy Lee's diagnosis had to take a number, had to get in line for priority in a list of calamities her life had become. Her father, her mother, and her cousin and close friend all died within a few months. Intimations of her own mortality did not get her full attention that year. She took the route suggested by her surgeon—a lumpectomy followed by radiation—and got on with dealing with everything else happening in her life.

When I was diagnosed, I knew very little about breast cancer, the disease, and a lot about breast cancer, the monster. I was transfixed by its press reports and adrift in misinformation. In those early post-diagnosis days, I was unable to separate the effects of the cancer and the side effects of the treatment; I thought breast cancer caused baldness, and I was fairly certain I would be dead in six months. At my first appointment with the surgeon, he drew a diagram of the lumpec-tomy he was proposing and wrote down the name of my cancer. I clung to that bit of paper, a crumpled talisman that went with me everywhere, because the drawing suggested that there were boundaries beyond which he would not cut. It gave me ridiculous comfort in its suggested possibility of containment that contradicted the dreaded word "invasive" in the medical term for my cancer: "invasive ductal carcinoma."

When the surgeon said, this is what I recommend, and the oncolo-gist said, this is what I recommend, I said, okay. I did not want a second opinion. Friends suggested I go to Toronto and talk to doctors at the Princess Margaret Hospital, where they knew about cancer; the underlying message was that in Ottawa, they didn't. This terrified me. I did not want to face the possibility that there was any uncertainty, any possible debate, about the way to defeat this disease. I simply wanted to be told the right way, so I could follow it. My first step on the treatment trail was as definite as Nicole's but for different reasons.

I acted out of determined ignorance; Nicole's decision was formed out of knowledge and experience.

When Laura G. was diagnosed, she embarked on another route. She questioned every step of the way. Her inquiries were informed by her own research and experience, as well as by her own clear ideas of what she would and would not be willing to do on this journey. She was 59, healthy and fit, with no breast cancer history in her family and had had her daughter at an early age; the usual risk factor suspects didn't seem to apply. She did grow up on a farm though, just outside Windsor, and research is now suggesting that farm women are nine times more likely to get breast cancer than non-farm women.[2] She remembers her father spraying the fields around their house with a special pesticide issued after the Second World War, made from leftover military supplies. He wore protective clothing and a mask. No one else did. So maybe there were environmental factors at play here? Who knows? What she did know is that she now had breast cancer and it had come out of the blue, a horrible, life-disrupting shock. "I've got a problem," she said when she phoned. "We're facing a problem." She tackled the problem the way Houston dealt with the accident-prone Apollo 13 mission. Full flat out. She was looking for a safe re-entry into her old world from which she'd been propelled by breast cancer.

The first surgeon Laura consulted recommended the standard approach: a lumpectomy, lymph node excision and, depending on whether the cancer had spread to the nodes, chemotherapy, followed by five weeks of radiation.

It was at this point that Laura took control. She did not say okay. She said, well, no, first of all, I am very clear about chemotherapy. I will not take it. The surgeon respected her decision. Second, she said, I do not want the nodes taken out. The surgeon wasn't quite so comfortable with this request. It made sense to Laura though. Since node removal is a diagnostic procedure to stage the cancer and guide treatment, she felt that such invasive, possibly debilitating surgery was unnecessary because she had already made her own decisions about what she would and would not do. She'd set her own parameters. She didn't need a sketch from a doctor.

Laura is an example of the modern patient, not willing to fall in line and do what the majority do without knowing why. She does her homework, thinks the issues through for herself. "I need information to make decisions," she says, "and they will be *my* decisions."[3] She is willing to expend hours of energy to try to find answers. Then, armed with articles and results of internet searches, "I beard the doctors in their dens," she laughs.

And that is very tiring because, at least in Laura's case, and hers is certainly not unique, there are always more beards, more dens, and seemingly more barriers. Some doctors feel overwhelmed by such a patient; they don't have time to deal with the questions, to explain why the drugs or procedures the patient has just read about in a magazine are not available yet and may never be; they don't have time to put out the fires started by loony internet information. Other doctors welcome such patients. An oncologist in Moncton, New Brunswick, says that informed patients "make it easier for doctors because they are more knowledgeable about what we are talking about, what we recommend." He allows though that when patients get hold of "premature" information on treatments that are not yet standard forms of therapy, it is often hard for these patients to accept why they can't have those treatments.

When Patricia Hurdle was diagnosed, she already knew far too much about breast cancer; she was no stranger to its pain and unpredictable behaviour because both her mother and sister had died of it. "I've been living with breast cancer since I was 12," she says softly. "That's when my mother showed me the lump in her breast."[4]

Then she overheard her mother and aunt talking late one night; the cancer had spread everywhere. Her mother had a radical mastectomy and then "she had cobalt treatment I guess it was in those days, and I remember her throwing up, and my father saying, 'Go help her' and I'm like, 'What can I do?'" What Patricia did was throw up too. Her mother died on her sister's birthday.

Patricia not only knew the disease, she knew the conventional—the gold standard—treatments, and she was highly doubtful about any success to be achieved by them. Her sister "did all the routine things: she had a lumpectomy, node dissection and radiation," Patricia says, "and [the cancer] came back and so she had a mastectomy and chemo and then she had massive metastasis . . . some people said this was *because* of the treatment, not in spite of it. . . . I talked to an oncologist in the United States at the National Cancer Institute, and he said, from his experience, chemo can bring on a 'shower of metastasis'. . . . So I was very skeptical about conventional treatment."

She went to see Bill O'Neill of the Canadian Cancer Research Group (CCRG) in Ottawa to discuss options other than the standard. O'Neill started CCRG in 1993 to provide information to cancer patients who felt they weren't getting the straight goods from their physicians. He later branched out into providing access to alternative cancer therapies not readily available in Canada and now offers alternatives directly to clients. O'Neill brings a passion to his work; he knows the frustration and fear of patients and their families newly thrust into a system that can seem so cold and impersonal. He is outspoken, adversarial and committed. His critics call him Dr. Hype and claim that he endangers patients' lives by luring them away from evidence-based treatment; his defenders call him Dr. Hope, a man who gives patients the most valuable commodity of all—a belief that they can and will get better.

Patricia says, "The medical system instils fear, and fear, and fear, and urgency to act . . . Bill was a good counterweight to that. He said, 'Look at other options'; he opened my mind despite the terror. The terror was the worst; to make any decisions in terror, it was a mistake, I realized. He said '[the cancer] has been there probably eight years, take your time, clear your mind.'"

Patricia did look at all the options and in the end elected to follow at least the first step of the treatment protocol suggested to her: a lumpectomy. Even though this was what her surgeon had recommended from the outset, now it was her decision. And she was comfortable with it. Like Laura, however, she chose not to have a node excision, though for a different reason. Her sister, who had died of breast cancer just four months before Patricia's diagnosis, had had node excision. Eleven nodes were removed—and there was no cancer in any of them. "So I didn't think there was any point," Patricia says.

"I hadn't decided yet whether I would do chemo or not." She stops and gestures around her to walls painted salmon pink; a soft, warm, healing room. "That's partly why I created this space—I thought I was going to be sick for a long time [from chemo] because the doctors said 'Do it all'; because of my family history they wanted to bring out all the guns." But "all the guns" had not helped her sister. Patricia made her choices based on the searing experience of watching her sister do all the "right" things and die within five years of what the diagnostics said was stage 1 cancer.

❧

The search for the cause of cancer is an intellectual pursuit—at least compared with the search for a cure—indulged in by cancer patients at idle moments. Definition of idle moments: after the initial terror of the diagnosis and before choosing treatment; between chemotherapy sessions; after chemo and before radiation; after surgery and before chemo; after radiation and before chemo; after a primary breast cancer and before a recurrence or metastasis. After metastasis, the whole exercise becomes less and less relevant. But the search for a treatment that is going to rid you of the disease, the delving into the witch's brew of treatments, touted or trashed, deciding which to choose, which to eschew, choosing whom to believe, whom to reject—this search is not of the brain so much as of the heart; it is visceral, immediate and all-consuming.

Treatment. We say "treatment," the books call it "treatment," but in our hearts, "treatment" means "cure." We are on a hunt for a cure. The treatment train hurtles us out of our old lives and into a new and terrifying terrain of statistics, choices, pain, hope, recovery and, sometimes, death. Susan Sontag, in her book *Illness as Metaphor,* calls it the "kingdom of the sick," where illness reigns as "the night-side of life." "Sooner or later," she writes, "each of us is obliged, at least for a spell, to identify ourselves as citizens of that other place." I especially like "at least for a spell." I like the hope offered in that phrase, that there is a way out of this place, that you don't have to take up permanent residence, that you could just be down there on a visit.

Each of us travels this new land in our own way. Despite admonitions from experts, friends and family, there is no wrong way, there is only your way. Second-guessing can kill just as fast as a cancer cell. Second-guessing yourself, that is, after you've made choices.

Some of us scramble for information, go for second, third and fourth opinions, question, challenge, research, take notes, make files, weigh and judge before deciding on a course of action. Others of us, some in a kind of paralysis of will, others through conscious choice, just do exactly as we are told by the first surgeon, oncologist or radiologist we see. Some of us move very, very fast; others take time to consider the options. There is nothing wrong with any of these approaches, as long as it is your way and not another's being imposed on you.

The treatment recommendations and options offered to us—to accept or reject—are based on an assessment of the stage of your cancer.

STAGING

After surgery, but before any adjuvant therapy, your cancer is staged. This imprecise science tries to determine if the cancer has spread, which is perhaps the most important thing to establish after a diagnosis. Breast cancer only kills if it moves out of the breast, which we don't need to survive, into vital organs, which we do. Susan Love, with typical honesty, titles her chapter on staging, "How We *Guess* if Your

Cancer Has Spread." She points out that there is no test or scan that reliably indicates metastasis and that doctors rely on circumstantial evidence to decide on the best treatment.[5]

The first step, a kind of pre-staging, starts with the surgeon even before a biopsy is done. He or she looks for swollen (palpable) or matted lymph nodes in the armpit and near the collarbone, palpates and assesses the size of the lump and checks the breast for telltale symptoms— puckering or dimpling of the skin, or whether the cancer has ulcerated through the skin. The next step is a more invasive investigation: a surgical biopsy of some sort.

Following a positive biopsy result, the next steps are, usually, surgery (either a mastectomy or lumpectomy) and the removal and examination of the lymph nodes (glands) from the nearest armpit to determine whether the cancer has spread from the breast. Called lymph node excision or axillary dissection, this procedure also reduces the likelihood of the cancer returning in the underarm. The surgeon cuts out a chunk of fat from the armpit in which are usually embedded at least 10 to 15 nodes. (The numbers vary depending on the person. One woman, Marcia Frank, had the standard-size scoop of tissue removed. It contained 27 nodes—all positive.) The pathologist checks the nodes; the number of positive ones are used in the staging of the cancer, which in turn dictates treatment options.

A less invasive technique is the sentinel lymph node biopsy. The surgeon injects a tracer element into the breast at the site of the tumour. This could be blue dye, a radioactive tracer or both. The theory is that the tracer moves naturally into the lymph system to the first draining node for that area, following the same trail as the cancer cells, if they have spread. This sentinel node is like the canary in the mine, not dead but blue or radioactive. If the pathologist finds cancer cells in this node, it is probable that there is cancer in others. If the sentinel node is clear, presumably a full node dissection is not needed. If it is cancerous, the surgeon removes more nodes to discover how extensive the spread is.

There is some controversy about this procedure. Clinical trials so far suggest that if there is no cancer in the sentinel node, there is a less than 10 percent chance that cancer will be found in others. However, in 2008, results of a long-term analysis of this procedure injected a note of caution: US researchers inone study found that one in four patients whose sentinel node biopsies declared them free of cancer were not. The biopsies had missed micromatastases — tiny cancer remnants that later developd into full-blown cancer. Another scary scenario, rare but possible, is that the sentinel node is packed with so much cancer that it does not pick up the tracer. Should this procedure be used in every case or just with those women whose lumps are smaller than a specific size? Surgeons don't agree. Should it always be done along with full dissection? Surgeons don't agree.

There is agreement in one area though. Make sure your surgeon is very experienced in doing sentinel node biopsies; the procedure is difficult to learn. The cryptic advice in the guide for patients and physicians published by the Canadian Medical Association is, ask questions, lots of questions, of your surgeon, because "surgical specialists who have not performed a large number of these biopsies may have a high failure rate."[6] It's been estimated that a surgeon must do 20 to 30 procedures before becoming good at it.[7] Dr. Roger Roberge, a breast cancer surgeon in Moncton, agrees: "Sentinel node biopsies are mostly still in [clinical] trials and should remain in trials [unless being done by doctors] who are doing a lot of this surgery. . . . I've been doing them for two years. I went to the Moffat Center in Florida and took the course and then [worked] in phase 1 trials, where we did the full dissection as well to see what percentage [of success] we had."[8] In two years, Dr. Roberge and his colleagues found only one positive node following a negative sentinel node.

The sentinel node biopsy has been added to the Canadian Clinical Practice Guidelines for the Care and Treatment of Breast Cancer (2001), and is more readily available across Canada outside trials.

Laura G.'s first challenge was to find a surgeon who would under-take to do the procedure at all, let alone one with lots of experience.

After her diagnosis in May, Laura was sent to a surgeon almost imme-diately. She worried about how quickly the appointment had been set up. But as Susan Love says, "Don't be scared by the word 'surgeon'—the fact that you're going to see a surgeon doesn't automatically mean an opera-tion. Surgeons are the doctors best trained to diagnose breast problems."[9] In Laura's case, it did mean an operation—her surgeon recommended a lumpectomy with lymph node excision. Laura rejected the lymph node excision without hesitation: "I'm not about to risk getting lymphedema by having all those lymph nodes removed. Especially when I will not take chemotherapy anyway, whatever is found in them."

Lymphedema is the swelling of the arm caused by an impaired lymph drainage system, which sometimes is the result of lymph node removal. The condition can be temporary or permanent, mild or extremely painful. It occurs less often now because of improved surgical techniques, but still, it is no laughing matter. As Love says, "Lymphedema has been vastly underestimated by the medical profession. The difficulties of women with lymphedema, physically and psychologically, are enormous."[10]

Nicole Bruinsma developed the condition two years after her surgery; it started slowly but became more and more painful and debil-itating. She wore an elastic bandage, "a compression sleeve" that fit her arm from wrist to shoulder. Good compression sleeves are usually custom-made and should be replaced every four to six months. "Do you know how much these things cost?" Nicole asked in indignant amazement. About $400. But it didn't help much: at times her arm was swollen to three times its normal size, throbbing and very painful.

When Laura G. told her surgeon she did not want the full lymph node excision, he did not mention the sentinel node biopsy alterna-tive. She asked about having just the lumpectomy with no nodes removed. He said that he did not do lumpectomies without node dissection. "He was gracious and friendly, but he wouldn't swerve from the standard approach," Laura says. "He pretty much kissed me off then, politely, of course." It took Laura eight months to find a surgeon who would do a lumpectomy without node excision.

Laura's experience with the system is not unique. If you want to step outside the guidelines, you are not always discouraged from doing so, but you may find yourself slipping into the interstices of a crumbling, overtaxed system. Doctors don't have time to help a woman navigate outside the channels marked by the buoys of the national clinical guidelines for breast cancer or by the clinical trials, whose objective is not to steer the patient into a safe harbour but to test the tools they give her to get there. You can be left without formal guidance. However, it appears that today oncologists and surgeons are at least more polite than a few years ago in accepting their patients' wishes to stray from the prescribed treatments.

⚯

The traditional staging classification, the TNM system looks at the size of the Tumour, the number of lymph Nodes with cancer in them ("involved") and whether the cancer has Metastasized. It goes likes this:

Stage 1: tumour is less than 2 cm, with no lymph nodes involved, and no metastasis

Stage 2: tumour is less than 2 cm, with positive lymph nodes (1 to 3); or 2 to 5 cm in size with either positive or negative nodes; or larger than 5 cm with no positive nodes, and no metastasis in all cases

Stage 3: tumour is very large with positive lymph nodes

Stage 4: tumour is large with positive lymph nodes and obvious metastasis to distant parts of the body.

It helps to know about these stages because you will hear them mentioned often—by your surgeon, your oncologist, your radiologist and other patients. It also helps to know that they are simply a way to try to establish treatment options, based on an imprecise statistical base built over the years. Most important to know is that the statistical prognoses these stages generate are out of date, preceding many advances in treatment, including the use of chemotherapy as standard adjuvant therapy. And then it helps to forget about them, because all they do is scare you if the prognosis indicated for your stage is not good. For every woman who fits into the prescribed statistical categories, you will find another who doesn't.

My cancer was stage 2 (small lump with two positive nodes). Not good. "Approximately 50% of patients with palpable breast cancer will prove to have axillary lymph-node involvement at surgery (pathologic stage II). These women are at high risk of subsequent systemic relapse and death from metastatic breast cancer, even though investigations at the time of diagnosis, such as routine blood counts, liver function tests and chest radiographic examinations, may reveal no evidence of cancer."[11] At the time, this stage put me into a 60 to 70 percent category for recurrence within five years. I totally blocked this piece of discouraging statistical prognosis—in fact, I often flipped it, putting myself into a more comforting 40 to 30 percent likelihood of recurrence. A woman I came to know was diagnosed at the same age and within a couple of months of me; she had the same treatments at the same cancer clinic for the same stage cancer. Within two years of her initial diagnosis her cancer came back; she had one treatment of Taxol (a particularly strong chemotherapy), which very nearly killed her, developed Bell's palsy and died within a few months.

This is because size and node involvement are only part of the story. When Carole LeBlanc found a lump in her breast, she wasn't too alarmed, nor was her doctor. She was 31 years old, living in Toronto, and had just had a miscarriage. "My doctor said, 'Don't worry about it; you are too young, you don't smoke, you're not on the pill, you just had a miscarriage so you are lumpy, your hormones are way high.' So I left it at that."[12] Carole was determined to get pregnant again, which she did six weeks later. The lump was still there, but because of the doctor's reassurances, she didn't worry about it.

After the baby was born, she and her husband moved back to Moncton. At her annual physical, her new doctor was not so sanguine. The lump was now really big. Carole describes that day: "She said that she was sending me for a mammogram and then an ultrasound; I said, 'Okay, when do I come back?' and she said, 'Well, no, we're doing them both today.' I knew then something was going on." And so did the radiologist, who sent Carole to a surgeon.

"I remember making jokes about it with my friend: 'I can just hear people back in [the small town Carole is from]—poor Carole, a five-and-a-half-month-old baby and probably dying.' I was making jokes out of it because *never* did I expect it to be cancer, never, because I was young, there was no cancer in my family, I felt great, I was never sick. . . ."

The needle biopsy came back negative, but the surgeon recommended a surgical biopsy to remove the whole lump. However, when he cut into the breast, the lump was so big, he left it, closed up the incision and told Carole "the news" as soon as she came out from under the anaesthetic. She had to have a full mastectomy.

After her surgery, the oncologist came into her hospital room: "'It doesn't look good; you will need chemotherapy.' They thought it had spread because of the size of the lump, so the treatment was going to be aggressive even though they hadn't even had the [pathology] results yet." But when Carole went for her first chemotherapy treatment, the nurse said to her, "Nobody called you? You don't need to have chemo." "Everything was clean, lymph nodes were clean, they were totally surprised," Carole says, laughing with delight at the memory. The size of the lump had completely misled them.

Other more accurate ways are being used now to try to establish how aggressive a tumour is, how fast it grows. An aggressive tumour can double every 10 days, a slow indolent one could take 20 years to double and so never become a problem in a woman's lifetime.[13] A pathologist will look at how many and how fast the cancer cells are dividing, how wild looking ("poorly differentiated") they are, the nuclear grade (the nucleus of the cell is the part that divides, so the grade indicates the degree of growth) and how odd-looking the nuclei are, whether there is cancer at the margins of the lump and surrounding tissue extracted, how many blood vessels are around the tumour (at a point in their development, tumours need their own blood supply and secrete something that makes blood vessels grow) or how much necrosis (dead cells) there is, which indicates whether the tumour has outgrown its blood supply, a sign that it is growing fast.

Other staging indicators have been getting attention recently. One indicator theory is that the location of the tumour can be a clue to prognosis. A study of more than 35,000 Danish breast cancer patients found that women whose tumours were on the upper lateral side near the underarm have a 15 to 20 percent better survival rate than women whose tumours are on the other side or lower on the outside.[14]

Biomarkers are moving quickly to the front of the line in breast cancer staging. These are certain biochemicals, the molecules of which indicate disease—indicators other than those that can be seen under the microscope that give clues to the characteristics of a tumour. Apparently there are a bunch, and the list keeps growing, but researchers still don't know which are the best, which will fulfill their initial promise. The ones you'll probably hear about most often are estrogen and progesterone receptors; tests are done to establish if the tumour is sensitive to these hormones and thus responsive to hormone-blocking or hormone-eliminating therapies. Tumours without hormone receptors (tumours that are hormone-negative) are more often found in premenopausal women and have a slightly worse prognosis than hormone-positive tumours, which are generally slower growing and are responsive, in most cases, to hormone therapies such as tamoxifen.

Another marker test that has received a lot of press in the last few years is the one that looks for too many copies of the Her2Neu oncogene receptor. (An oncogene is a tumour gene that, when triggered, transforms normal cells to cancer cells.) Her2Neu is one of the dominant oncogenes that contribute to cancer, and its overexpression indicates an aggressive tumour. It also turns out that it can be used to indicate what might be the best treatment for a particular cancer.[15]

Some researchers have found that the levels of the protein cyclin E indicate whether early breast cancer is likely to metastasize. The announcement of the astonishing accuracy of this protein as a cancer marker ("six times more powerful a predictor than tumour size and lymph node involvement") was accompanied by the usual caution of the scientists involved, belying the glaring optimism of the media headlines: "The results might not be as impressive in a bigger study."[16] Other researchers described the results as intriguing but also cautioned that they had to be confirmed through additional studies and longer follow-up of patients. Science gives, and science takes away.

STANDARD TREATMENTS

It is no wonder the military metaphor reigns in the corridors of cancer treatment when the three major therapies—the slash, poison and burn trio of surgery, chemotherapy and radiation—all trace their roots to war. Although the first surgeons were barbers, surgical refinements (cutting in such a way that the patient didn't immediately bleed to death or die of shock) were developed on the battlefield. Chemotherapy was born out of chemical weapons, and radiation therapy was thrust into a lead role on the medical stage as "the sunny side of the atom" after the bombing of Hiroshima and Nagasaki in 1945.

After I had surgery and the results of the node excision indicated that the cancer was on its way through the lymph system, my oncologist said, "This is an aggressive cancer, and we have only one kick at the can. We have to hit it hard." Hitting hard meant using the direct assault approach, the weapons of mass destruction.

Surgery

Surgery is a local treatment, its goal being to remove all the cancer in the breast, even if cancer cells have already moved from the primary site. The surgery could be a lumpectomy (removal of the tumour and a margin of tissue around it) or a mastectomy (removal of the whole breast). It is difficult to assess success in the broad spectrum of surgery —with or without adjuvant therapy—over the last decade or so, but we've certainly come a long way since the days when few women survived the procedure, especially before the use of anaesthetics. The first recorded use of ether for removal of a tumour was not until 1846. Before then, you got to chew on a mandrake root perhaps or you might have been given a few belts of wine before going under the knife. As surgery, including amputations, became more common in later centuries, patients were encouraged to get thoroughly plastered before the operations, in an effort to dull the pain.

In 1879, it was reported that out of 143 women who had had a radical mastectomy in England, "a mere 35 survived for any length of time at all."[17] At about the same time, an Austrian surgeon reported on the outcome of 170 operations he had performed between 1867 and 1876. He was attempting to prove that cancer, contrary to the claims of the doomsayers, could in fact be cured with the knife. The doomsayers might have had a point. Whatever spin you put on it, the stats were not encouraging: only 4.7 percent of the women operated on were alive three years later.[18]

The famous Halsted mastectomy, introduced in the 1890s, became the surgical treatment of choice for the next 75 years. William Stewart Halsted, an American surgeon, believed that removal of the breast, all the lymph nodes in the nearest armpit and the chest wall muscles would contain the cancer. The underlying premise was that cancer remained in the breast for some time before spreading, and that the lymphatic system was relatively separate from blood vessels, so removal of lymph nodes would prevent the passage of cancer cells.

The popularity of the Halsted mastectomy among surgeons persisted even in the face of research as early as the 1930s reporting that an identical percentage of women survived after less severe surgery; equally good results were being achieved with lumpectomies followed by radiation.[19]

By the 1970s, it was accepted that tumours could not be cut out by their roots like weeds and that removing lymph nodes did not deter the spread of cancer because the blood and lymph systems are so integrated. However, the Halsted continued to be performed well into the 1990s in North America. It still is in some places.

Still dominating the surgical scene is the 20-year-old debate about which is more effective, lumpectomy, also called breast conserving surgery (BCS), or mastectomy. Research published in 2002 found there was no difference in the survival rate of women who had a mastectomy and women who had a lumpectomy with radiation. Lumpectomies may be more effective now because surgeons pay more attention to the importance of ensuring "clear margins": in performing a lumpectomy, if they suspect that there are cancer cells in the tissue around the lump, they do a wider excision to try to "get them all." If in doubt, go wider.

Dr. Monica Morrow, a breast-cancer specialist at Northwestern University, wrote in the *New England Journal of Medicine* that "it is time to declare the case against breast-conserving therapy closed," and that this research should convince "even the most determined of skeptics."[20] It won't. The debate will continue as long as breast cancer continues to mystify. It is truly horrifying to many women who, when told they have breast cancer, are informed at the same time that they can either elect to have the whole breast removed, or just the lump and margins. It is not an easy decision.

The Canadian Clinical Practice Guidelines for the Care and Treatment of Breast Cancer offers this advice in answer to the question, "Do I have a choice between mastectomy and lumpectomy?: Yes, in most circumstances. There is clear evidence that lumpectomy, when followed by radiation therapy is just as effective as mastectomy. . . . Since they are equally safe, the deciding factors are often your own personal preference and circumstances, as long as the cancer is in the early stages. For most women, lumpectomy is now the recommended procedure."[21]

Now the recommended procedure. Today, the studies indicate there is no difference in outcomes; tomorrow, the studies may show something different. In the meantime, it is up to you. What seems to be the sensible route here is the one that most doctors and the guidelines recommend: find out the pros and cons of each procedure for your specific situation, decide what you are most comfortable with, talk to your doctor, listen to your heart and make your choice. Easy to say. But at present, all the research in the world is not going to make it any clearer, unless, of course, one or the other route is obvious in a specific case. For example, a very large, aggressive tumour in a small breast would suggest a mastectomy; a tiny non-invasive lump would suggest the lumpectomy route.

A new procedure on the horizon, currently in clinical trials at the M.D. Anderson Cancer Center in Texas, is one involving high-frequency radio waves that can literally cook the tumours from inside. Using an ultrasound for guidance, the surgeon inserts a multipronged probe into the lump. The prongs open up and melt the cancer cells without burning healthy tissue.

Other techniques being tested include blasting the tumour with heat from lasers, microwaving them and freezing them to death with injections of argon gas (a method called cryoablation). These are all in clinical trials and several years away from being available as standard treatment options.

With new visual tools, cancer surgery has become more precise. Tiny fibre optic cameras now relay images to a monitor and new versions of MRIs let surgeons operate while the 3-D images are taken. There are also new versions of ultrasound and CT scans.

Chemotherapy

Most histories of cancer therapies attribute the discovery of modern chemotherapy to an explosion on a ship carrying mustard gas in 1943. Often described as a "serendipitous" event, it launched medical researchers down a new path, soon to become one of the busiest highways in cancer treatment. Chemo's provenance serves warning that it is more a weapon than a therapy. The word itself simply means the control of a disease or condition through drugs—Aspirin is technically a chemotherapy. The word was coined in 1907 by chemist Paul Ehrlich, who mused about the "magic bullet," the hypothetical drug that would eradicate a specific disease, just as the plants promised in Cherokee lore.[22]

The accident on the ship wasn't serendipitous for the sailors who died from breathing the noxious gas unleashed by the explosion. But the results of their autopsies were. They showed that the chemical had killed off the fast-growing cells of the bone marrow, a discovery that led to speculation that it might kill off other fast-growing cells, such as cancer cells. An industry was launched. The challenge ever since has been to find drugs and establish dosages that will kill the cancer without killing the patient too—the magic balance. Chemo is the perfect illustration of 16th-century Swiss physician Paracelsus' adage, "The dose makes the poison."

Chemotherapy, a systemic treatment, reduces the risk of breast cancer recurrence by one-third. When I first heard this, on a TV documentary, I thought, wow, that sounds like a pretty good argument for chemotherapy. But a third of what, I then wondered. Author Susan Love does the numbers for you; turns out, it is not quite so straightforward as it might seem. The claim of "one-third" is a proportional reduction rather than being across the board, which changes the impact of that claim dramatically: "If you have a 60 percent chance of recurrence, a one third risk reduction means it will reduce it by 20 percent but if you have a 9 percent chance of recurrence the one third reduction in mortality is only 3 percent."[23] And the numbers become even less significant once you know that they are based on another set of numbers to do with risk assessment, which are proving to be as unreliable as the weather. Yet, a survey of oncologists indicated that they rated the probable success of chemotherapeutic treatment at three times higher than was warranted.

Research published in 2002 suggests that chemo offers no benefit for post-menopausal women with hormone-sensitive breast cancer that has not spread to the lymph nodes. This reinforced an earlier study, begun in 1988, that found the survival rate was the same for women with tumours under two centimetres with no node involvement whether they had chemo or not. So you have to be careful when weighing the risks and benefits, because what we do know about chemotherapy is this: there are hundreds of chemotherapies, there are dozens of combinations used (coyly known as "chemo cocktails"), there is the current gold standard treatment, which gets upgraded or downgraded as the efficacy of other drugs are compared with it in clinical trials. Currently the taxanes are the frontrunners—Taxol and Taxotere—but as is the case with all chemotherapies, their effects vary from patient to patient. Their high toxicity has killed some women before the disease could; other women have benefited from these drugs, which seem to have slowed disease progression dramatically.

Some chemotherapies are administered intravenously and some are given orally; most have nasty side effects (nausea, hair loss, heart damage, nerve damage, immune system damage). The collateral damage is because chemotherapies are not "smart bombs," though researchers are working on that; they destroy all fast-growing cells, not just cancer cells, and that's the big problem. Chemotherapy is the very opposite of smart; it's like a big, stupid bully let loose in your body, swinging out wildly, smacking everything in its ken. The goal is to haul it out of the fight after it flattens the bad guys but before it wipes out the whole schoolyard.

Radiation Therapy

Radiation therapy is almost always used in conjunction with surgery. Doctors talk of using the treatment to "mop up" cancer cells that may have escaped the knife. "Mop up" sounds pretty benign. Don't be fooled. This treatment is not benign, but it has come a long way from the early days when cobalt was used as the source of radiation. Many women I spoke with described their mothers' experiences—burnt and blackened flesh and open suppurating wounds caused by such early treatments.

Mary Trafford's mother had radiation treatment for breast cancer in 1971. She had a recurrence in 1993, and three years later was admitted to the hospital with a variety of complications, mostly gastrointestinal problems. During one of the medical tests, her heart stopped beating. The doctors told Mary that the radiation her mother had had for her breast cancer 25 years earlier had damaged her heart, causing problems all these years later.

Radiation machines now use electricity as the radiation source, which provides sharper beams (less scatter area around the target) and lower dosages. The angle of the beamed radiation is more precise, hitting mainly breast tissue, and less likely to hit vital organs (heart and lungs), as was the case 20 or 30 years ago.

Statistics indicate that the local recurrence rate of breast cancer following a lumpectomy and radiation is 10 percent, compared with 35 percent for a lumpectomy without radiation. But it comes at a price. It is still an insidious treatment, one of the clues being that if you have had radiation once, you cannot have it again to the same area—too much damage has already been done there. Short-term effects can include fatigue and skin damage ranging from a "slight sunburn" to much more severe burning. I was warned of the "sunburn" effect but ended up with a weeping wound that took several weeks to close. (Turns out I might have avoided this by eating curry. Tests on mice have found that curcumin, the compound that makes turmeric yellow, reduces blistering and burns from radiation treatment.) However, side effects vary from person to person. A friend who had radiation three years ago said her skin barely reddened from the treatment. She did not suffer from depression, a side effect common immediately following the treatments. I went into a deep blue funk for months, and this was long before I knew it was a fairly common after effect.

If you have had the lymph nodes removed from the armpit, radiation can compound the damage already done there by surgery; it can worsen the nerve damage into your arm and it can increase your risk of lymphedema.

Another long-term problem to watch for is skin cancer. If you have had radiation treatments, it's a good idea to have a dermatologist check both the entry area and the exit area (on your back) from time to time. Skin cancers such as basal cell carcinoma and the far more serious malignant melanoma can result from radiation treatments.

One of the most depressing aspects of radiation treatment is its length, usually 25 to 30 consecutive sessions. However, recent research (2008) indicates that a lower total dose of radiaton delivered over fewer sessions can be as effective as the standard approach. Another recent development is IMRT (Intensity Modulated Radiation Therapy), 3-D conformal therapy that is also often administered over fewer sessions (see introduction). Radiation implants are being used at some centres and for some cancers rather than external beam radiation. A form of brachytherapy, which has been in use for some time for prostate cancer, this five-day treatment plants radiation "seeds" in and around the tumour site. This is not always offered instead of the 25 to 30 sessions, though. After Laura G.'s lumpectomy, her radiologist recommended both: the implant method as a mopping-up after the beam method, which was mopping up after the lumpectomy. That's a lot of mopping up.

When the surgeon discovered that Laura G's tumour was very close to the chest wall, he was worried about the lack of clear margin; in fact, he wanted to go back in and do more cutting. Laura demurred. She was strongly encouraged to have radiation but was told that the beam would have to be angled deeper than usual to ensure coverage of the tumour site. When she asked about possible damage to any organs, the radiologist said that her heart would not be affected but her lung might be. "As long as you are not an athlete, you won't even notice." Cold comfort.

Laura cast around for an alternative.

This trio of therapies has held sway for decades, usually in a lockstep of surgery, chemotherapy and radiation, although the order sometimes is switched and the last two sometimes, though rarely, administered concurrently, depending on the specifics of the case.

When you look at the big picture, it appears that progress has stalled at this point because this same trio is still the main offering at the treatment table. My breast cancer was diagnosed in 1988. The first-line treatment recommended for me was the same as that which has been recommended for 25 or 30 years, with some minor variations: surgery, chemo and radiation. I didn't know then that many oncologists, surgeons and radiologists, as well as most epidemiologists, were quietly despairing of those treatments: "Thirty-five years of intense effort focusing largely on improved treatment must be judged a qualified failure."[24] And yet.

Nicole was diagnosed nine years after I was. Same regimen of treatment for her primary cancer, but with a stronger, more toxic chemotherapy. A close friend received her diagnosis in 2007: the base treatment on offer? Surgery, chemotherapy and radiation, only difference was that chemo came first. These are the three therapies featured in the Canadian Clinical Practice Guidelines for the Care and Treatment of Breast Cancer, updated in response to research literature reviews conducted every six months.

Although researchers are exploring new directions, clinicians are still primarily using toxic and invasive treatments. In 1996, *Scientific American* reported that for the top 12 types of cancer, including breast cancer, surgery, radiation and chemotherapy were still *de rigueur*. This is still true today. And it will be, it appears, tomorrow. In approximately 375 cancer-targeted drugs currently being studied in clinical trials, 175 of them are "anti-cancer"—a euphemism for toxic and invasive. (Cynics might say that part of the reason for their continued use is the big bucks involved: the worldwide "anti-cancer" market was projected to be near US$30 billion by 2003, nearly double what it was in 1998.[25])

Proponents claim that there *is* progress with this trio, that it's in the "minor variations." "Minor" is relative, however: if you are a patient at the receiving end, looking down the barrels of surgery, chemotherapy and radiation, the variations seem infinitesimal; you are still the target of the big guns, the blunt instruments. That they have been refined over the years is not immediately evident. For some physicians, for scientists, and ultimately for us all, though, these refinements are significant. Dr. Richard Margolese from the Jewish General Hospital in Montreal says that the survival rates from 1900 to the late 1980s didn't change much. But since the 1990s, there has been a significant improvement in all parts of the Western world, "and that's because of the combination of the small advances we've made, and we need to pile advance upon advance and make slow progress in that way."[26]

However, the "small advances" of each of these three treatment modalities seem to be moving in tandem with a development that is not particularly comforting to patients: the ratcheting up of the standard versions of each to stronger, more invasive, levels. Surgeons are carving out larger margins around a tumour; radiation, although lower in dosage than a couple of decades ago, in some cases is now intensified with the teaming up of beam and implant radiation sessions; and tough chemotherapies, such as the taxoteres, which had been reserved for the treatment of metastatic disease, are now being used to treat primary breast cancers. In an article entitled "New Hope for Cancer," Dr. Larry Norton, a medical director at Memorial Sloan-Kettering Cancer Center in New York, says, "I think there is no question that the war on cancer is winnable."[27] But this same article places progress blithely on the shoulders of harsher chemotherapies, reporting that "the risk of recurrence" was "significantly" reduced by "simply replacing one of the standard chemotherapy agents with a drug called docetaxel (Taxotere)." The word "simply" is the clue that the writer has never had to have chemotherapy.

Often when you ask about progress in chemotherapies, the answer sidesteps, referring instead to the success with the medication administered to quell chemotherapy's side effects. There is measurable progress with anti-nausea medication, which is much more effective than it was even a few years ago. One problem, though, with the new drugs that control side effects so well is that doctors don't know when to stop treatment. It's very difficult to find the tolerance level, because the body's messages are being muffled.[28]

It's more difficult to measure whether chemo itself works. Defining "works" is the first problem; depending on the stage of the cancer at initial diagnosis, depending on whether it is primary or metastatic, depending on the age of the patient, and so on, usually 5-year or 10-year survival are the benchmarks. In a sense, this is totally meaningless. You survive the breast cancer for 5 years, and one day later, you die. Did the chemo "work"?

The second problem is resistance. A drug or combination of drugs might work for a while, but eventually the cancer cells build up resistance and continue on their merry way. "The history of cancer therapy is that the cells are much smarter than the clinicians, and [they] quickly evolve pathways that can bypass the treatment."[29]

So, answers to direct questions about progress in chemotherapies over the last decade seem either shifty, despairing or positively bizarre. My favourite is this one: "Like many medical treatments, chemotherapy has not attained complete perfection." However, "not everyone survives cancer, but almost everyone survives chemotherapy."[30]

Maybe it's an impossible question to answer. I asked one oncologist, working in cancer treatment for more than 30 years, if he thought chemotherapies were getting any more successful. His response started out confidently. "Certainly," he said, with just a touch of impatience at my question. "Yes, there's been a lot of progress in chemo. It has had an influence on outcomes." He paused for a minute, then continued, less certainly: "A modest improvement but nevertheless an improvement. . . ." He went on to talk about the importance of clinical trials:

"[they are] a sequential process and they take time, comparing one treatment to another to another to see which is the most effective." He talked of the process, not the result. He talked of success in comparative terms, one treatment over another, but not about what patients want to know—an answer not in terms of degree but in terms of absolute. Not whether one drug is better than another but whether any are any good, period. No one can answer that. And I felt kind of mean trying to get him to. His honesty disarmed me. "Is chemo the answer?" he said, this man who has administered chemotherapy for a long lifetime—his—to countless patients, in good faith, in fervent hope that he was helping them fight off their cancer. "Is chemo the answer? I don't know." What he did know was that the new directions in breast cancer treatment were real progress; here something was very much "working."

5 TREATMENTS OF INDIRECT ASSAULT: THE STEALTH ATTACKERS

One of the discouraging things the public, and patients in particular, face is the continued and repeated promises of the magic bullet that never really arrives. It's important for us to be more straightforward about this, that there won't be a single magic bullet but there are tremendously promising things coming forward. What it's going to take, however, is an appreciation of what the targets are in a cancer cell and aiming at multiple targets—we can't kill a tumour cell simply by taking out one of its legs, we've got to knock all its legs out from under it.

—Dr. Gerald Batist, Jewish General Hospital, Montreal[1]

AFTER SHARON HAMPSON'S SECOND GO-ROUND with cancer, she was put on tamoxifen, a hormone therapy. "I took it for five years," she says.[2] Then one of her doctors told her to come off it, that it was not safe to stay on it longer than that. But another of her doctors disagreed, telling her to continue taking the drug. "'I've had patients on it for 20 years, and there's been no problem," he told her. "Always conflicting advice, always," she says resignedly. "It takes a huge emotional toll."

98

For Sharon, it is a toll heightened by a sense that she had become earmarked as a troublemaker. "Do you think there is a note on my file or something, saying this woman is a shit disturber? I do speak up for myself," she says. "But it's not without a price."

It is a roller coaster ride, both because of the disease and because of "all the other stuff—it eats you up," she says, "the stuff around the edges." Not just the worry about being labelled a troublemaker because she asks questions and won't be sloughed off, not just the fear generated by false diagnoses, but the uncertainties around the treatment for the real ones.

Breast cancer treatment has seen a big shift with the advent of hormonal therapies (not to be confused, which I did for many years, with hormone replacement therapy [HRT]). As seems to be the pattern in the history of medicine, this new arrival was looked on with suspicion and at first had to slug it out with proponents of chemotherapy, who ruled the castle in the late 1970s. However, over the years, they've joined forces, and in the quartet of mainstream treatments, chemo and hormonal therapies play the leads now, with surgery and radiation in ancillary roles,[3] although I'm not sure that the order matters to a woman who is encouraged to have them all. But hormonal therapies represent, in at least one respect, a huge advance. They did not rise up from the flipside of weapons developed to kill. They are not the blunt instruments of frontal attack; they don't slash, poison or scorch; they infiltrate, they block, they impersonate, they work behind the lines. They are the more subtle fifth columns of the war against breast cancer.

Hormones are simply chemical substances produced by various glands in the body; they circulate via the bloodstream and cause effects in other tissues. There are lots of hormones, but the ones you hear about most often in relation to breast cancer are the female sex hormones: estrogen, which is produced by the ovaries, adrenal glands, placenta and fat; and progesterone, produced in the ovaries during the menstrual cycle (not to be confused with progestin, an artificial hormone sometimes given to post-menopausal women as hormone replacement; the drug Provera is an example of progestin).

The belief that estrogen promotes breast cancer has been around for a long time and is now well established, though only relatively recently has it given rise to attempts to control the disease by decreasing hormonal stimulus.

In the staging of a tumour, one of the most important pieces of information is whether it is hormone dependent. If it is, it is thought to be more responsive to a range of new hormone blockers called SERMs, or selective estrogen receptor modulators—selective because these drugs in some instances block estrogen and, in others, actually act as estrogen. The SERM you probably hear the most about is tamoxifen, which has been used as a cancer therapy for more than 20 years but originated in 1967 as a fertility drug. Tamoxifen acts as an estrogen-blocker in the breast (but acts as a weak estrogen in the liver, hence, the descriptive "selective"). Although it can cause blood clots and uterine cancer, it is considered almost a miracle drug in the treatment of breast cancer. Women on tamoxifen have fewer recurrences and 30 to 50 percent fewer cancers in the other breast. The big controversy about tamoxifen is not in relation to its use in *treating* breast cancer but in its use in *preventing* it—as chemoprevention.

HORMONAL THERAPIES AS PREVENTION

Prevention. Oh boy, this term has opened a Pandora's box in recent years. It became the bandwagon in the late 1990s, with everyone from researchers to fundraisers to the media leaping aboard. But, it turned out, everyone had his or her own interpretation of the term, and the bandwagon careened wildly through the literature and the conferences, scattering confusion and anger in its wake. "Prevention" became a catch-all for a range of measures. "High resolution mammography, blocking estrogen with tamoxifen . . . and genetic testing followed by a preventive double mastectomy went holus-bolus into the mix with research on dietary fat, reducing alcohol consumption, and eating broccoli."[4] It became clear, with the approval of the National Surgical Adjuvant Breast and Bowel Project P-1 Study (NSABP, the Tamoxifen Breast Cancer Prevention Trial), based in Pittsburgh, Pennsylvania, that the bandwagon was being steered into the spongy and controversial territory of medical intervention as a prevention measure.

The Tamoxifen Breast Cancer Prevention Trial involved 13,388 women at increased risk for breast cancer. Women were eligible to enter the trial if they had a 1.7 percent or higher risk of developing the disease in the next five years, which is considered double that of the average North American woman. Under this definition, all women over the age of 60 were eligible, as were women in their 40s with one or more first-degree relatives with breast cancer and a personal history of at least one benign breast biopsy or a diagnosis of lobular carcinoma in situ. This is a huge range of women to be considered eligible for medical intervention for a disease they do not have.

It was the first time such a powerful and, indeed, not fully tested drug, with known toxic effects and known to be a carcinogen—since one of its side effects could be another cancer—was given to a healthy population. Adriane Fugh-Berman, author, physician and chair of the National Women's Health Network, said the trial was a dangerous precedent because it blurred the crucial demarcation between disease prevention and disease treatment, "which are two completely different fields, and that's the way it should be."[5]

On the other side of the argument are those who, along the lines of "It's a small price to pay," believe that it's preferable to prevent breast cancer with a comparatively benign drug than have to treat it with the full arsenal after it blossoms. Because tamoxifen apparently has fewer side effects than does chemotherapy, at least at the time of its ingestion, it is looked upon as the lesser of two evils; in fact, as Sharon Batt, breast cancer activist and author, says, it is promoted in the American media as if it were no more threatening than a vitamin pill. However, consider the following answers to the question, "What are the risks of taking tamoxifen?"

- Impact on Fertility. Tamoxifen may affect fertility, so it is important to use some form of birth control while you are taking this medication. However, do not use oral contraceptives (the "pill") since they may change the effects of tamoxifen.
- Blood clots. Women taking tamoxifen may have a slightly increased risk of developing blood clots in the lungs or large veins. This may be especially true for women undergoing chemotherapy (anti-cancer drugs) while taking tamoxifen.
- Stroke. Women taking tamoxifen may also have an increased risk of stroke.
- Endometrial cancer. Tamoxifen may increase a woman's risk of developing endometrial cancer (cancer of the lining of the uterus). . . .
- Cataracts. Taking tamoxifen appears to put some women at increased risk for developing cataracts. . . . People have also reported eye problems such as corneal scarring or retinal changes.[6]

Doesn't sound like any vitamin pill I know.

The North American prevention trial was launched with great fanfare. In 1998 it was ended early with equal fanfare because its sponsors deemed it so successful that they claimed it would be unethical to continue to give the control group in the trial a placebo: their preliminary findings indicated that tamoxifen reduced the incidence of the disease by 49 percent in high-risk women.[7] The same results were not found by two European trials, which concluded that there was little or no reduction.

"The possible reasons for the differences in results have been the subject of much discussion, but no clear explanation is available," say the authors of the report from yet another trial, the International Breast Cancer Intervention Study (IBIS), published in 2002. "Three clinical trials on the use of tamoxifen to prevent breast cancer have reported mixed results. The overall evidence supports a reduction in the risk of breast cancer, but whether this benefit outweighs the risks and side-effects associated with tamoxifen is unclear."[8]

Their study, which involved 7,000 high-risk women, suggested a reduction of breast cancers by about one-third (though some experts questioned the validity of this claim because it included in situ cancers) but also indicated that tamoxifen "significantly increased risks to health and life." Women on tamoxifen were two and a half times as likely to get life-threatening blood clots—43 women in a group of 3,500.

The commentary published in *The Lancet* accompanying the IBIS trial report sums up the dangers of chemoprevention: "A cardinal requirement of chemopreventive agents is that they must be safe. Because they are given to many people, most of whom will not get the targeted condition, the agents must have a low profile of adverse effects. Tamoxifen clearly does not have a safety profile that would allow it to be used by enough women to have a large impact on the overall incidence of breast cancer. Here the IBIS trial adds a new concern about tamoxifen: an increase in all-cause mortality. . . . Most disturbingly (and unlike the previous studies), the IBIS study also reports a significant increase in the total number of deaths in tamoxifen-treated women."[9]

At the time the North American trial was called off with such hoopla, Dr. Bernard Fisher, one of the trial directors, was asked in a CBC TV interview if tamoxifen could be causing an increase in the incidence of uterine cancer. He responded, "Will the ceiling in this room fall down? We don't know the answer."[10] The results of subsequent studies are suggesting that the ceiling is starting to show cracks. A higher incidence of uterine cancer is showing up among women who are taking tamoxifen.

In the meantime, AstraZeneca has been marketing the drug under its trade name Nolvadex for the prevention of cancer in healthy women in the United States. The wording allowed by the Food and Drug

Administration (FDA) in 1998 was that tamoxifen could "reduce the risk of breast cancer in the short term but could not prevent it."[11] In interviews at the time of the FDA ruling, an oncologist and spokesman for AstraZeneca was contemptuous of what he viewed as semantics and pointed out that the FDA could not dictate what doctors might say to patients in their examining rooms. A disturbing development since then is that a change in the American drug laws allows pharmaceutical companies to advertise prescription drugs directly to the public. This isn't legal in Canada yet, although there are indications that it might soon be, but of course Canadian women and their doctors are exposed daily to tamoxifen advertisements through the American media.

Health Canada has not approved tamoxifen for the *prevention* of breast cancer, but it is prescribed in this country for the *treatment* of breast cancer. However, through a loophole in Canadian drug laws (known as "off-label prescribing"), physicians may give it to healthy women at their discretion.[12]

Dr. Richard Margolese, a strong proponent of chemoprevention, sees this direction as very much the way of the future: "If I had to give you a theme for the next decade, it's prevention," he says. "The disease is not cancer; the disease is carcinogenesis. If you think about it, cardiologists don't wait until there is a heart attack, they look at the cholesterol and the blood sugar and the blood pressure and they try to prevent the heart attack. That is the complication. Cancer is the complication. The process that leads to cancer, which we now can identify, is the disease and we need to treat it with drugs like tamoxifen and other drugs that we are searching for. . . ."[13]

Another high-profile SERM is raloxifene (manufactured by Lilly and sold as Evista). On the market since 1999, it was initially used as a treatment for osteoporosis. Raloxifene was thought to act in the same way as tamoxifen, blocking estrogen from reaching estrogen-receptor-positive tumours and it appeared to have a slightly better track record in preventing recurrences or metastases.

It was also being tested as a prophylactic for breast cancer. In 2002, the authors of a Clinical Practices Guideline discussion wrote: "Although the raloxifene research is promising, questions concerning treatment duration, side effects and overall mortality are as yet unanswered. These may be answered by the Study of Tamoxifen and Raloxifene (STAR) conducted by the NSABP, which will compare the effectiveness of the 2 drugs in preventing breast cancer."[14] The questions have been answered but absolutely not conclusively (see introduction).

If chemoprevention is to be accepted as a viable intervention, then research must offer evidence that it leads to a reduction not just in breast cancer incidence but in breast cancer mortality rates. As well, "newer drugs that have a better safety profile need to be developed. Finally, better ways are needed to target the drugs to those women who will benefit most. Current risk-assessment tools are inadequate for this purpose."[15]

This sums up the three major issues here. First, at this point, there is no evidence that chemoprevention reduces the numbers of deaths from breast cancer, although it appears that it does reduce the incidence of breast cancer. Second, the drugs currently offered to prevent breast cancer are not benign, underlying the difference between acceptable risk for someone trying to avoid the disease and someone who already has it. And third, the biggest issue, how can a woman's risk for developing breast cancer be accurately assessed? The answer, at present, is that it can't be. Or as the Canadian Task Force on Preventive Health Care and the Steering Committee on Clinical Practice Guidelines for the Care and Treatment of Breast Cancer so gently puts it: "The assessment of a woman's baseline risk of breast cancer presents challenges for physicians."[16]

THE DIFFICULTIES OF ASSESSING RISK

One of the most commonly used assessment tools for breast cancer risk is the Gail index, which, based on certain risk factors, including age, age at first period, family history, and ethnic background, "estimates a woman's risk for invasive breast cancer over the next 5 years and her lifetime risk and compares her risk to that of a woman of the same age who has normal risk factors."

For women at low or normal risk of breast cancer (the Gail index sets this at less than 1.66% at 5 years), the recommendation is that they should not take tamoxifen to reduce the risk of breast cancer because "the data from the randomized controlled trials are conflicting, a reduction in breast cancer mortality has not been demonstrated, and the harms from tamoxifen reported in other similar trials outweigh any benefits in this low-risk group."

For women at higher risk of breast cancer (Gail index puts this at 1.66% at less than 5 years), the recommendation is that this group be counselled "on the potential benefits and harms of breast cancer prevention with tamoxifen." The cutoff for defining high risk is arbitrary but "examples of high-risk clinical situations are 2 first-degree relatives with breast cancer, a history of lobular carcinoma in situ or a history of atypical hyperplasia."[17]

The experts do agree on one thing: the need to know what you are letting yourself in for if you choose chemoprevention. The Canadian Clinical Practice Guidelines for the Care and Treatment of Breast Cancer as well as the US Preventive Services Task Force recommends counselling for high-risk women on the risks and benefits of taking tamoxifen as prevention.[18]

It appears that many women consider taking tamoxifen based on nothing more than a free-floating worry about getting breast cancer, rather than on their real risk factors.[19] This worrisome development suggests that women don't recognize the dangers of ingesting a toxic drug in the same manner as a vitamin pill, an attitude encouraged by direct-to-consumer advertising now permeating the popular media.

NEW DIRECTIONS IN TREATMENT

In the treatment area, other hormonal therapies are showing promise, including the aromatase inhibitors. Aromatase is the enzyme responsible for much of the estrogen in post-menopausal women. About two-thirds of post-menopausal women with breast cancer have aromatase in their breast tissue, giving the breast its own supply of estrogen.[20] The theory is that by blocking this enzyme, the amount of estrogen is drastically reduced. One of the first of these drugs—Arimidex (the brand name for anastrozole)—is showing promise, as is Aromasin (exemestane) and particularly Femara (letrozole) in the treatment of metastatic disease, after the cancer has become resistant to tamoxifen. In October 2003 a large Canadian-led international study of letrozole, chaired by Paul Goss, at Princess Margaret Hospital in Toronto, indicated an astonishing 43 percent reduction in the risk of breast cancer recurrence. The study involved 5,187 post-menopausal women, all who had been on tamoxifen for five years after their diagnosis and treatment of their original cancer. In an eerie echo of the tamoxifen prevention trial, this study was halted early because the study team felt that it would be unethical to continue giving the control group a placebo. However, within days of the announcement, the criticism and cautions began. In particular, there is concern that because the study was ended after only two and a half years, the long term safety and efficacy of the drug cannot be determined.

The use of monoclonal antibodies, a gene-based therapy, is also garnering attention. These drugs target certain proteins in cancer cells to block the tumour's ability to absorb the growth factors researchers believe regulate cell proliferation and oncogenesis. Herceptin (trastuzumab) is the first of these gene-based therapies, which goes after the Her2Neu protein, produced in some women with breast cancer. The key word here is "some." The initial euphoria about this therapy has been tempered by its relatively narrow application, since only about 30 percent of women with breast cancer have an overabundance of the protein.

In one area of research, viruses are the unlikely allies in attacking cancer. They've been given the trendy title of "smart bombs" because they are being harnessed to attack specific targets. Normally, a virus works by finding its way into a cell, where it replicates until the jam-packed cell ruptures and dies, releasing the virus into the rest of the body. Researchers are attempting to genetically alter viruses to target cancer cells and avoid healthy ones. In the meantime, Canadian researchers have discovered reoviruses, which are naturally harmless and target only cancer cells.

Then there are the "stealth" molecules. Here again, military terminology dominates: researchers at the Mayo Clinic have patented a "genetic bullet" that "targets, then shoots down, proteins needed for disease."[21] Known as "anti-sense" molecules because they lock onto the messenger RNA and make no sense to other parts of the cell, these molecules appear, so far, to work on rats.

Other research is focusing on therapies that cut off the blood supply to a tumour. To continue growing beyond the size of a small pea, solid tumours need their own blood supply to survive and thrive. To do this, they carry out a process known as angiogenesis: they secrete substances to stimulate blood vessel growth in neighbouring tissue and induce these vessels to grow new branches in their direction. The anti-angiogenesis drugs being developed and tested, unlike chemotherapy or radiation, are designed to shrink, not destroy, tumours by starving them of blood.

Vaccines are also being studied. Researchers are experimenting with dozens of different vaccines, some (autologous) built from the cell-line of the individual to be treated, some built from "generic" cancer cells. As with any vaccine, the goal is to provoke an immune response in which the patient's white blood cells attack the cancer cells but not healthy cells.

All these therapies can get truly confusing because there have been so many developments in the last decade or so. Current cancer treatment research is like Stephen Leacock's rider, the fellow who jumped on his horse and rode off in all directions: toxic drugs to blast the cancer to oblivion, gene therapies that slide in and tinker with the DNA, anti-angiogenesis drugs that cut off the blood supply and starve the cancer to death, immunotherapies that don't attack the cancer directly but provoke the immune system into taking care of it and drugs that block hormone stimulation. As Dr. Batist says, there is no single magic bullet. What we need is a barrage of bullets, a range of different therapeutic approaches, because it seems that while a single attack might take off one of the tumour's legs, it is busily growing others.

The accepted wisdom is that knowledge is power, but with its infinite variety, the torrent of information about therapies can render you power*less*. Because it's early days yet for many of these therapies, it's impossible to assess progress in the short term because of the two-step dance of early research: one step forward, one step back. This can be thoroughly unsettling when you are one of the dancers. For example, an hour's trawl on the internet netted the following: "New cancer drug shows early promise." Reading further, you discover that this drug, in the anti-angiogenesis stable, is so new it doesn't have a name, has been tested on only 23 people, and reduced tumour size in 6 of those patients. Next story: "Innovative breast cancer therapy tested on Vancouver Island." Called radiofrequency ablation (RFA), it is a process whereby a small probe is inserted into the breast tumour, opening up like a tiny umbrella to deliver radio-frequency waves to zap the cancer. It is in clinical trials on 22 women. Next story: "Switching off gene kills cancer, study finds. In what researchers are calling a huge and unexpected finding, scientists report they have been able to kill cancer by briefly deactivating a single gene." Reading further, you find that the scientists are talking about mice. One of the oncologists who wrote the study says cautiously, "It is a conceptual breakthrough," and researchers warn that it should not be confused with a "near cure."[22]

Dr. Linda Penn, a researcher at the Ontario Cancer Institute, says, "A new wave of therapeutics is coming down the pike, and it is an exciting time to be a cancer researcher."[23] It is too, but it's a discouraging time for doctors who are caught between the promising theories and models of science, and the realities of the front-line treatment centres.

Such wilting promises are even tougher on patients, especially those with advanced disease, where time is running out. Novelist Carol Shields, who died of breast cancer in 2003, made just this point in a sly inclusion in a comment made by one of the characters in her novel *Unless:* "Injury, when it comes, arrives from so many different directions that I don't even attempt to track it. News from Indonesia or Jerusalem. Bush heating up for the election, breakthrough advances in cancer research—"[24]

What happens is that you read all the hype and headlines about a new therapy, for instance, Herceptin. You go to your doctor, full of hope that it will help you. And your doctor has to tell you that since you don't have the Her2Neu protein, it is a non-starter for you. The articles you have read have omitted that pertinent fact. Or you're slated for radiation therapy and you are dreading the 25 consecutive days of treatment. Perhaps you don't live near the treatment centre and figure you will have to stay in the cancer lodge or with a relative or friend. Then you read about a new approach in a magazine you are flipping through as you wait to see the doctor. The article says that after a lumpectomy, a tiny radioactive bead is planted right into the tumour site. Treatment takes "a matter of days, not weeks," it says. Hopes up, you ask your doctor about it. "Would this work for me?" He points to the fine print: "Clinical trials on 70 patients nationwide have been completed. The procedure is waiting approval." It might work for you, but it's not on offer yet.

You might be told you are at high risk for breast cancer and that you should be taking tamoxifen as a preventative. You know about the controversy concerning the practice of prescribing tamoxifen for healthy women, and you've been unnerved by the most recent findings that although tamoxifen does reduce breast cancer incidence in high-risk women, it also "significantly increases risks to health and life." What to do?

Then you read about the broccoli pill. Researchers at the University of Illinois have designed a chemical compound based on a naturally occurring anti-cancer agent found in the vegetable. Double bonus: not only do you prevent cancer, but you don't actually have to eat broccoli. You ask your doctor about it. He's bemused. He's never heard of it, asks where you found out about it. On the internet. Oh, the internet, he says despairingly. He offers to find out more, and at your next visit reads out the line you missed: "Tests on mice have shown promising results." In other words, don't hold your breath. As Scott Findlay says, "Mice aren't humans: we would have cured cancer 50 years ago if they were."

THE DICHOTOMY OF STANDARD TREATMENTS

It's important, and often difficult, to remember the distinction between standard treatments—those recommended most often by most doctors—and therapies that are in their infancy, still swaddled in research and cautious optimism, taking baby steps out of the labs via clinical trials. The standard treatments are the ones you will hear about most often in the doctors' offices. They are the ones described in the Canadian Clinical Practice Guidelines for the Care and Treatment of Breast Cancer, revised versions of which are released by the Canadian Medical Association. Canada was the first country in the world to publish a patient-friendly, plain-language version of such medical texts. It provides, in question-and-answer format, easy-to-understand information on the various stages of investigation of a lump through to treatment options. It is very much the mainstream, which is both its strength and its weakness. These guidelines provide comfort in their clarity, organization and authority. They reflect what you will probably hear from your doctor. What they can't do is provide specifics, options or customized advice. Dr. Kathleen Pritchard at the Toronto Sunnybrook Regional Cancer Centre cautions that the guidelines are there "to set a basic standard for the diagnosis and treatment of breast cancer. Doctors and patients may want to deviate from them for very valid reasons."[25] A dichotomy exists here: how do standardized treatment guidelines operate at a time when researchers and physicians are saying that breast cancer may be not one but many diseases and that variations might depend on the individual? Dr. Pamela Goodwin, of

Toronto's Mount Sinai Hospital, says, "We believe that 10 years from now we will be able to look at the precise characteristics of a breast cancer in an individual woman and prescribe therapies that target exactly the tumour that she has. . . ."[26]

A Toronto biotech company, Arius, is using a patient's tumour material to develop an antibody tailored to attack his or her particular cancer; the drug will be custom-made for each patient. This isn't a new approach, but it does seem to be one of the ways of the future. "The principle [behind the research] is that everyone is different," the founder and president of the company, Dr. David Young, says. "With current cancer therapy, it doesn't matter who you are, because if you fit a certain profile, you'll be treated that one way." The theory behind the Arius model is that each person's cancer has a "fingerprint" or marker that triggers a specific antibody to attack it. At present, all users are offered the same drugs that may or may not work, Dr. Young says. "If the drug doesn't work you'll get all the side-effects without the benefits. . . ."[27]

Although the national guidelines do allow room for adjustments and alterations to be made according to the specific situation, critics believe that the guidelines encourage a cookie-cutter mentality and that some doctors will use them to rubber-stamp treatment without considering the specific requirements of their patients. Others think that the guidelines establish a kind of safety net below which medical advice and treatment cannot fall.

The situation is this: research (including clinical trials) forms the basis for treatment protocols that, since 1998, are written into the Canadian Clinical Practice Guidelines. Physicians rely on these guidelines as parameters for decisions on treatment for individual patients. Patients, understandably, expect the recommended treatments to work. After all, they are the gold standard. But they are the gold standard only in comparison with other treatments, not in relation to the ultimate goal of cure. They do not address—they cannot address—the unknowns. And it is the unknowns that cause the anguish in the front lines. When something goes amiss in the lab, when an expected result doesn't pan out, the researcher is disappointed, but rarely anguished. And he or she goes back to the drawing board. When the expected result doesn't pan out in the cancer treatment room, the physician and the patient often don't have the luxury of going back to the drawing board. As my oncologist said, "We have just one kick at the can, and we're going to kick it hard." If the can doesn't crumple, you can keep kicking it, and sometimes it flies off, and sometimes it defies the kicker, and sometimes the kicker misses entirely. It is the uncertainty of outcome that is so confounding.

In Moncton, breast cancer surgeon Dr. Roberge summed up the frustration so many physicians feel:

I had two patients, both aged 27, they both had the same first name, and I operated on both for breast cancer within one month of each other. Both had several positive nodes, both had massive chemo and had to go away for bone marrow transplants. This was about seven years ago. They don't do bone marrow transplants for breast cancer anymore except on rare occasions, but in those days we thought it worked. One of those women still runs with me in Run for the Cure in October; I see her every year, and in my office as well. The other one died within months. Yet they had very similar diseases, they had the same number of nodes, same kind of treatment, they were the same age, same everything. But for one, it didn't matter what we did, we couldn't get the disease under control; the other, as I say, is great. So there are a lot of unknowns. It's frustrating. Very, very frustrating. There is so much we still don't know.[28]

Just how much do we know? A whole lot more than 300 years ago, otherwise we'd still be cutting off breasts with a hot knife. A lot more than 50 years ago, when the arrival of chemotherapy and radiation brought a brief flash of hope that breast cancer was curable. It wasn't, but the knowledge accumulated about its workings, and the progress made in its staging allowed researchers and doctors to, in effect, divide it into two diseases, one "curable"—primary disease if it didn't come back—and one not—metastatic disease if the cancer came back in other parts of the body. Metastatic disease was not curable, because the cancer cells attacked and destroyed organs vital to life; primary breast cancer was, because the cells remained in an organ not essential to life. This was a semantic loophole through which crumbs of comfort could be thrown to women newly diagnosed. But it was like saying, you are safe from the barbarian hordes, as long as they elect to stay inside the barricades—when there are no barricades. This was progress though; not just a word game but an indication of a much deeper medical understanding of the disease at the cellular level.

And we know a lot more than even 15 years ago, when the breast cancer genes BRCA1 and BRCA2 were discovered and it seemed— for a few heady months anyway—that all we had to do to eradicate breast cancer, along with all other diseases, was to find the gene that matched and fix it. It would be like a game of Snap, with a deck of 35,000 cards: researchers would turn over every card against every disease and yell "Snap!" when they found a match. (With apologies to genetic scientists everywhere.)

Dr. Kathleen Pritchard of Toronto Sunnybrook Regional Cancer Centre says, "I can tell patients about therapies I didn't have to offer five years ago, about tests on their tumours I didn't have five years ago, and there will be a lot more of these in the next few years."

Dr. Pamela Goodwin of Mount Sinai Hospital says, "We have a whole host of new treatments for breast cancer. . . . We will be able to obtain better tumour control and perhaps even eradicate the tumours."

Dr. Gerald Batist of Jewish General Hospital says, "I am very optimistic about the treatment of breast cancer not only in the future but in the present."

All these doctors speak in the TV documentary *Reasons for Hope*.[29] The version I saw, in 2003, was a remake of a documentary shot four years before. The producers told me that the doctors had been re-interviewed for this update, and the same breast cancer patients appeared again. Except for one. She had died in the interval. The film opens with a shot of three women talking to each other: "Four years ago, these three women had the courage to share with us. . . . now they do it again . . . ," the voice-over says. "They are all healthy, happy and full of life." In the video copy I bought from the film's producers, there is no mention of the missing patient who isn't. Death has been edited out.

The world of breast cancer is littered with a number of necessary disconnects: between the domain of statistics and the reality of individual experience; between research and practice; between the critical imperative of optimism and the batter of failure. If you are told that you have stage 4 breast cancer, most physicians would encourage you to suspend belief in the gloomy statistical prognosis attendant on advanced metastatic disease, to disconnect from the very foundation on which your treatment options were built. Patients are reminded constantly of the huge gap between the lab and the front lines of therapy, encouraged to suspend not belief in this instance but expectation because the connection between the two, as far as it relates to their immediate quest, is as tenuous as a cobweb, a time-space continuum that is not to be relied on in their lifetime.

And a total disconnect is required to grasp, at the same time and with the same brain, the shiny optimism of claims of progress and the grainy realities of the disease, to connect the pronouncement of one speaker at a recent conference that "we are slowly moving toward the sun: we can and we will find the cure" and that of the next speaker, who answered her own question: "In this new century, regarding cancer, especially breast cancer, has anything changed? Yes, but not for the better." What trips us up is the kind of peculiar logic exercised by the research clinician who claimed that we did have a cure for breast cancer . . . as long as it didn't come back. It was as if recurrence were a different disease. Such thinking appears to allow for the coexistence of optimism and pessimism and the simultaneous assertions of successes and failures of breast cancer treatment.

ARE WE MAKING PROGRESS?

So just how are we really doing? That depends on who you ask and how you define progress.

Annie Sasco of the International Agency for Research on Cancer (IARC), World Health Organization, doesn't think so well, at least when you look at the global picture. In the world, there are 1,050,000 new cases of breast cancer each year; the incidence of breast cancer between 1980 and 2000 has almost doubled, an increase much larger than can be explained by the growing world population; there are 3.9 million women living with breast cancer: it is the number one cancer for women in the world, even in developing countries, where it has recently overtaken cervical cancer.

The picture does look better for mortality rates, at least in the industrialized world: more women are surviving longer—60 to 80 percent survive past the five-year marker. However, in developing countries, the picture is much bleaker. In Africa, only 10 percent of women with breast cancer live for more than five years.[30]

In Canada, the overall mortality rates for the disease have declined steadily since 1990: by 1997, the overall Canadian breast cancer mortality rate was at its lowest since 1950. In 2008, an estimated

- 22,400 women (up from 21,200 in 2003) will be diagnosed with breast cancer, and 5,300 will die of it.
- 170 men will be diagnosed with breast cancer, and 50 will die of it.
- On average, 431 Canadian women will be diagnosed with breast cancer every week.
- On average, 102 Canadian women will die of breast cancer every week.
- One in 9 women is expected to develop breast cancer during her lifetime. One in 28 will die of it.

Breast cancer accounts for almost one in three cancer diagnoses among

Canadian women, and 175,000 women have "first-hand experience" with the disease.

Those are the cold numbers behind which lie a lot of pain and suffering, fear and death.

Do these stats represent progress? We all put our own spin on them. The optimists focus on the fact that fewer women in Canada are dying of the disease; the pessimists say, yes, but more women are getting the disease.

There are a few indisputable facts: we are a lot better off now than 35 years ago, when the cumulative effect of the various treatments on offer was horrific: "After having the breast and underlying tissue on one side of her chest cut away and covered with a thin skin graft, a woman could be subjected to intense radiation therapy, primitive forms of chemotherapy, the removal of her ovaries and eventually, the removal of her adrenal glands. If this failed, she might be injected with male hormones that made her skin oily, pimply, and hairy."[31] The advent of hormonal therapy has done away with adrenal gland removal and works—at least for a while—in the treatment of metastatic disease, chemo is accompanied by more effective anti-nausea drugs and radiation dosages have been reduced. More lumpectomies are being performed. Early detection seems to be eliminating some cancers before they can spread.

Scientists at the Reasons for Hope Breast Cancer Research Conference in Quebec City in 2000 announced progress on several fronts. We were told that researchers were "poised in the doorway" of finding the cure for breast cancer; that we could "confidently look forward to when this disease is the thing of the past." Alan Bernstein, then president of the Canadian Institutes of Health Research (CIHR), said that "for researchers in the field of breast cancer, and for women and their families who are suffering from this terrible disease, there are more reasons for optimism now than ever before. . . . We are at the defining moment in understanding breast cancer." Twenty-five years ago, the breast cancer cell was a black box, he said. But now we know most of the secrets of breast cancer cells: how they work, what they will do. Now the challenge is to exploit that knowledge. "Over the next generation, we should get to the point when our daughters and granddaughters will ask us, "What was breast cancer?"[32]

Then the words of caution crept in: There is no cure around the corner, he continued. We have a long, long way to go. Which about sums up the ambivalence about the progress in treating this disease, the juxtaposition of wishful thinking with the realities. It's how you define progress: progress in the lab is one thing—all the mice don't die, that's progress; in the chemo rooms, the cancer wards, all the women don't die—that's not progress.

For a woman with breast cancer, true progress has to be defined as the development or discovery of a drug, a therapy, an approach that can be counted on, always, to slow or eliminate her disease. "Counted on," with no statistical hedging, with no waffling about redefining the disease as a condition to which we then bring different expectations, to prevent a primary cancer from becoming metastatic. This is not the case yet.

There is progress in what some call the "soft" areas. Soft doesn't mean unimportant; it refers to less tangible developments, the psychosocial issues that are harder to measure. Generally, the stigma of breast cancer does not carry the fearsome weight it once did, which means fewer women are keeping their disease a secret until it kills them. Women are better informed, willing to seek second opinions, eager to participate in decisions. Many have exchanged secrecy for action, and silence for sharing their experiences with other women in the same predicament.

6

PITY THE POOR PARSNIP: FROM THE LAB TO THE REAL WORLD

For months now I had been meticulously observing parsnip canker.
I had made copious notes. I had many specimens. But I could not bridge
the chasm between my long row of parsnips in the laboratory, all in
various stages of fetid death, and the remedy that might exist for all
this rotted vegetable flesh on the opposite shore of science. Or miracle.

—Helen Humphreys, *The Lost Garden*[1]

IN HER SEARCH for a surgeon who might do a lumpectomy without node excision, Laura G. was elated to find a doctor in Montreal who appeared willing to consider approaches other than standard ones. He recommended right off the bat that she start taking the aromatase inhibitor Femara. This was before he knew whether her tumour was estrogen-positive and would respond to a hormone therapy. And wasn't Femara usually prescribed for metastatic cancer, after the patient stopped responding to tamoxifen? This was puzzling. Laura took the prescription reluctantly but did not fill it: "This stuff costs $7 a pill, and I'm not even sure if I should be taking it," she said.[2]

119

When she returned two days later, the doctor gave her a sheaf of documentation for the clinical trial. Huh? What trial? "First I'd heard about this," she said.

She was in a quandary. She was there by herself, so had no one with whom to discuss this latest development: since she had no idea a trial was in the offing, she hadn't expected to be faced with any decisions at this appointment. The surgeon wanted a decision that day and she was having difficulty understanding him—both in French and English. The trial consent forms seemed to absolve everyone from everything that might happen to her, ever, and she didn't even yet know what was on trial. She was beginning to think it might be her. When she finally gleaned that it was for a new radiation procedure and not a drug, she signed. It didn't commit her to anything, just perhaps cleared the way, although she still wasn't absolutely sure for what.

"Turns out it was irrelevant anyway," she said, "because I was told I was not eligible—I didn't meet the criteria for this particular trial." Her tumour was too close to muscle and bone (it was within a centimetre) for this particular approach to be a viable option.

Femara, on the other hand, was still a trial possibility. In fact, Laura later discovered that there was a shortage of participants for the Femara trial. Perhaps this was why the doctor had been so eager for her to take the drug? She never did find out, and she still has not filled the prescription. Nor has she gone back to that doctor.

Nicole's experience was quite different. When the gold standard treatments failed her, and when alternative therapies failed her, Nicole and Scott searched the world for a clinical trial in which she might find something that would work. They both understood that the primary purpose of a trial was to test a drug, that its possible benefit for her was secondary. But now, this was just so much meaningless fine print. She had no other options. She needed something, and she needed it fast.

They heard about a vaccine trial in Amsterdam, but it did not have regulatory approval yet; it would be a long while before that trial got under way. Nicole didn't have a long while. Then they found out about a doctor in Chicago who had been using another form of vaccine on a small number of patients, apparently with promising results. But Nicole was turned away because the FDA had shut down the trial and no more patients could be put on the therapy.

Then their research turned up another promising lead: a clinical trial for metastatic breast cancer patients on a heat shock protein vaccine was to be set up at Sloan-Kettering, a research hospital in New York City. They went to Sloan-Kettering, only to find that the trial didn't even have a protocol yet (an outline of objectives, methodologies and admission criteria) and that recruitment was a year away. "This is no good for me," Nicole said. She did not have a year.

The Sloan-Kettering researcher told them of another trial, this time on polyvalent vaccines (made up of a combination of different antigens). Could Nicole be part of this trial? Well, she fit the protocol, but the trial was full. She could put her name on a waiting list though; she would be the 102nd patient on the list. They couldn't bring any more people into the trial until they found more companies to manufacture the vaccine. How long would this be? At least six months. "I don't have six months," Nicole said in despair.

Whatever route you choose to follow after diagnosis, you will certainly hear about clinical trials, where the worlds of science and medicine blur together like heat on the horizon. There is prickly debate about trials, but one thing is certain: in the current medical system, all roads to progress in breast cancer treatments lead through the valley of clinical trials, a road that bumps over a washboard of failures as well as successes, where individual participants can become unintentional sacrifices to science. It focuses on the age-old fine line between the good of the people and the good of the person.

When you are caught in the collision of the two worlds, the fallout can be devastating. Serving science is a siren song for some doctors, and when the good of all takes precedence over what you perceive as the good of you, it comes as a shock. I was caught unawares at a routine hearing test. I hadn't been checked for more than a year, my hearing was certainly worse in one ear and the tinnitus was a constant jumble of ringing, swooshing and twittering. Maybe when the doctor looked into my ear he would see a tiny flock of birds. But he didn't look in my ear. He just messed with my mind.

First were the hearing tests with the technician: tones, headphones, white noise, repeat the words after me. Then in came the doctor. As he read the results, I watched him, with just a hint of hostility because this was the doctor who had told me a few years before that I was socially unacceptable. He meant my hearing level was socially unacceptable, but that's not what he had said.

He looked up suddenly. "You have lost 50 percent of your discriminatory hearing in your right ear since your last test." He leafed back through my records (they go back years to when I first came to him for tests to monitor the family deafness that stalks us all).

"You've had carcinoma of the breast?"

"Yes."

"You had chemotherapy and radiation?"

"Yes." Realization dawned. "Are you saying this hearing loss could have been caused by treatment?" I was off and running. "Why can't doctors be more honest about after-effects of treatment? I have skin cancer from radiation now, and nobody warned me about that possibility." I had ratcheted up to a full-bore rant in seconds. "And when I was in treatment, my eyes and throat were affected, although the radiologist told me it was a summer cold, absolutely no connection with the fact that I was a nuclear test site for 25 days in a row, and everyone else I knew who was radiated for breast cancer had that same summer cold, no matter what the season. I'm beginning to wish I'd never had radiation."

"You can't do that," the doctor interrupted brusquely. "You must take the treatment modality that is available at the time. It is the best that can be offered until new studies are done. You must become a number, because this is a scientific environment and it is the only way we will discover better treatments. Double-blind studies. And then a thousand patients later we will have better treatments."

What was he talking about? I wasn't a number.

He went on, "And if I get prostate cancer, I will be a number too, a patient, not a doctor. That's the way it must work."

Astonishment momentarily silenced me.

"But I'm not talking about treatment," he said, and for a few seconds I thought he was reassuring me. "Radiation didn't cause this hearing loss. It's the cancer I'm talking about. It may have."

My hearing was suddenly working 100 percent. "You mean a tumour in my ear?"

"No, but it could be metastasis to the brain. Or it could be nothing. . . ."

When the subsequent scans and tests turned up nothing, I changed doctors. I figured he wouldn't mind, since I was just a number.

Nicole had a similar lecture from her oncologist when she was faced with metastasis. She described their conversation: "He mentioned that at this stage, my primary responsibility was to enrol in a clinical trial, as this was the only way we were going to find out the 'truth' about this disease. . . . He said, 'And I hope, Nicole, that someone in your position would encourage others to do the same.' This is to say that at the time of diagnosis of metastatic disease, you cease to be a *person* who has a life worth saving and suddenly become an *opportunity* for a data point in some study or other." She was blisteringly angry.

Clinical trials are where patients are brought into the labs and scientists into the cancer wards. It is no wonder this area can be so contentious when such a chasm exists between the aeries of pure science and ground zero of the disease, each with its own language, its own priorities and timelines, its own ethics and truths. The mix of the two worlds can seem like oil and water, especially if you are swimming in it. It is where we become the parsnips, the mice and the primates. At a research conference on breast cancer, one scientist inadvertently illustrated why the mix can be so frightening. In her presentation she spoke of what she called a particularly "beautiful" study in which "some primates were oophorectomized." The women in the audience sat straighter, listened more closely. Did she mean us? We are primates, right? Then she really made us nervous. Outlining another study involving rodents, she started talking about "These women . . ." She stopped and apologized with a nervous laugh.

There are the folk in the front lines: women and men fighting the disease at a purely personal level, and physicians helping them, explaining therapies, administering therapies, providing reassurance and comfort when the therapies don't work, cheering when they do— the human face of the disease. Away from the front lines, sometimes very far away, are the scientists who work in the slow, slogging, repetitive, methodological tasks of their profession. They are less concerned with the fate of individuals who have the disease than they are with the disease itself. And they must be; it is a necessary distancing, allowing for a different set of values, different methodologies to come into play. It allows for seeding mice with tumour cells, performing unnecessary oophorectomies on monkeys or painting parsnips with pesticides. It allows for the crucial checks and balances of science: the replication, duplication and verification by other studies and other researchers. For scientists this is the only way. For those in the front lines, it can seem just endless process when what we want is proof.

But in science there is no such thing as proof: "No matter how many times a theory has been tested, and found tried and true, there is always lurking in the background another competing theory, which is equally consistent with the observed results to date."[3] This is a tough concept for a layperson to hang onto, especially when you are also an individual hoping and praying for some scientific absolute that will solve the mysteries of your disease.

Clinical trials are exactly that: trials, or experiments, to test treatments in a clinical setting, where people are the guinea pigs. Sounds brutal and unethical, and in the past some of them certainly were. One of the most infamous came to light a few years ago in the United States. In rural Georgia in the 1930s, 400 African-American men with syphilis were given a placebo instead of medicine so that the doctors could study the progress of the disease. Some of these men survived and suffered for up to 40 years, the doctors watching all that time, never telling them what they had, never telling them they were going untreated, not even giving them penicillin when it was discovered and proved to be a cure for the disease. I thought, perhaps naïvely, that such abuses were in the past, that we were talking history here, until I read about an equally chilling study conducted by American scientists in Africa in the 1990s who "monitored, but did not treat the monogamous, uninfected partners of more than four hundred HIV-positive individuals for two and a half years. Nearly a hundred became infected during the course of the study."[4]

Such abuses notwithstanding, most clinical trials and studies nowadays are hedged with rules, rigid criteria, ethical guidelines and watchdogs, all in place to prevent such egregious practices and to arrive at credible findings via the ladder of the scientific method. Their purpose is to develop a drug or procedure that works better than those currently in use.

In the beginning is the hypothesis. Most of the time, anyway. It may surface in an orderly fashion from an observational study. Or it may rise out of a scientist's hunch. Scott Findlay knew about evolutionary resistance (his initial training was as an evolutionary biologist) and he had a hunch about how it might operate in the area of cancer treatment. "My research had nothing to do with oncology and all to do with ecology," he says. But when Nicole became ill, he started applying his knowledge to medicine and how the body's eventual resistance to chemotherapy could be countermanded. Scott hypothesized that an examination of resistance as an evolutionary phenomenon might provide some insight into treatment for cancer patients.

A hypothesis might blossom from a serendipitous event—such as the mustard gas explosion in 1943 that started medical researchers hypothesizing us into the golden era of chemotherapy—or from the discovery that a drug developed to treat one condition appears to have an impact on another. Raloxifene (Evista) was brought through clinical trials to the marketplace as a treatment for osteoporosis, but when it was observed that women taking the drug seemed to have a lower incidence of breast cancer, it was put into trials as a treatment for that disease; it is now one of the standard hormone therapies prescribed for breast cancer.

A hypothesis also might be born backwards out of empirical evidence of something for which there is no theoretical explanation. A general example of this would be the neo-catastrophism theory of climate change. Ice scientists in Greenland cored down thousands of feet into glaciers and came up with disturbing evidence of abrupt changes in climate; not gradual global warming, but apocalyptic changes. Hypotheses didn't send them searching for this evidence; the evidence sent them searching for hypotheses, just as the empirical evidence of anticipatory nausea many women suffer *before* their chemo launched a rash of hypotheses to explain the phenomenon after it was observed.

A hypothesis may start with one scientist or a team of scientists, but when it is flung into the tough, exacting arena of research, it gets smacked around by other scientists trying to knock it out of the ballpark. Researchers at the Reasons for Hope breast cancer research conference did just this to the "diagnosis by hair" theory. In 1999, a group of scientists reported in *Nature* that an abnormal ring visible in X-rays of a hair could be used to diagnose both the existence of breast cancer and the susceptibility to it. Other scientists said, "Well, we don't *think* so." Actually, they said, "Although the data strongly supported the conclusion, any underlying cause for the correlation seemed hard to fit into our current understanding of breast cancer. We set out to replicate the original findings using a blinded, qualitative and quantitative approach."[5] They found no consistent relationship between breast cancer and hair structure. That will not be the end of it though. Other scientists will look at other hair and come up with other conclusions.

The most orderly arrival of a hypothesis is from observational studies. Cross-sectional studies accumulate data by asking a large group of people about a specific symptom or topic at a specific time, such as asking women if they feel sick before each chemo treatment in a study of anticipatory nausea; "case control" studies compare groups of people who are similar in all but the one aspect being studied, for example, comparing women who have been on HRT for 10 years with women who haven't to see how many in each group developed breast cancer. The third category includes "cohort" or follow-up studies, such as the BSE studies in China and Russia, which tracked a large group of women for several years to see if breast self-examination was effective in early detection.

A hypothesis, let's say, about a drug that seems to shrink breast tumours in mice, could languish in a lab for years, at the level of basic research and animal testing, before breaking out into a clinical trial. Or it might leap sideways out of other research into the cancer treatment centres full of people, not mice.

Phase 1 of a clinical trial studies the safety and tolerable dosages of a drug or therapy; this is its sole purpose, reflected in the fact that less than 5 percent of subjects in phase 1 trials get any health benefit whatsoever.[6] But most patients don't realize this and are convinced that there is therapeutic benefit for them.[7] Depending on the stage of their cancer, for some it doesn't matter; their reasoning is that they have nothing more to lose, except their life, which they are losing anyway.

About 30 percent of phase 1 studies don't make it any farther. Phase 2 studies look at the effectiveness of the drug, based on the dosages established at the phase 1 level. Phase 3 trials compare the drug being tested with the standard therapies (the gold standard). Typically, there are three arms of a phase 3 trial: the drug being tested, and two others or combination of others in current use. Placebos in phase 3 cancer treatment studies are rarely used, particularly in chemotherapy trials. However, chemoprevention trials for women at risk for developing breast cancer do include placebo.

Phase 4 trials look at a drug or therapy after it is in the marketplace.

Most oncologists are very much in favour of clinical trials; one told me why. "I am a believer in scientific methodologies for medical protection regarding a drug or product," he said, "and in the last 50 years, that has become a very elegant form of studying drugs in a very scientific way; you find out how they work and their benefits, and therefore you know, as a doctor, what you are doing and why you are doing it. You know what you are giving to your patients."[8] Eventually. Within a randomized trial, it could be that neither you nor your doctor knows which drug you are getting. What you are assured of is that whatever treatment you get, it is not expected to be less effective than the one in current use.

You hear the unsettling terms "randomized" and "double-blind" to describe these trials. Randomized simply means that patients are randomly assigned by computer to one or other arm of the study: you can't choose which. Nor is your doctor supposed to be able to. Double-blind means that neither you nor the researchers know which drug you are getting. These controls are in place to prevent biased results; they are crucial to the research component of the trial that, in keeping with the scientific imperative, must, rightly, perceive participants as parsnips; they have nothing to do with the medical—the human—side, the individual medical situations of the people in the trial.

This highlights a dangerous misunderstanding of clinical trials, not so much in how they are set up and conducted, though that is also a point of contention, but in how they are presented to, and perceived by, patients. The goal of clinical trials is to test a product or procedure. The participants, the subjects, are the tools in this process. How they fare is important to the researchers as data points—numbers—that are summarized into statistics to guide the next trial, or point to the next gold standard. How they fare, on a personal level, is not the concern of science. And that's another tough concept to handle when you are either encouraged to go into a trial, or when you are desperately seeking one that will accept you.

INFORMED CONSENT

Before you can be enrolled in a clinical trial, your doctor must establish that your situation meets every one of the eligibility criteria, and must explain the true objectives of a trial and outline the risks involved—the very nature of human testing obviously involves risk. Then you must sign consent forms acknowledging that you understand everything you've just been told. According to Health Canada, "ethical standards require that participants in a clinical trial be fully informed of the potential risks and benefits associated with the drug, as well as the availability of alternative treatments. This process, known as informed consent, ensures that the participants are aware of their rights, as well as their responsibilities within the study."[9]

Unfortunately, participants are usually not in receiving mode at the time they are asked for their "informed" consent. Most often, the forms are presented to you while you are wreathed in the fog of post-diagnosis terror, a time when you could hardly take in a newspaper headline, let alone up to 30 pages of single-spaced, badly photocopied legalese. It is so easy to misunderstand.

These forms are documents that seem to absolve everyone from the hospital board members to the maintenance staff for anything that might happen to you in the trial. Many participants don't realize that clinical trials are conducted mainly to benefit future patients, not themselves, that the treatments being tested are not yet proven to be better than the current standard therapies. They also might be riskier, with tougher side effects. These "therapeutic misconceptions" are common among patients, even after they've signed informed consent papers asserting that they fully comprehend the pros and cons of the clinical trials. What is possibly more worrisome is that many doctors harbour the same misconceptions. One study found that, "to the researchers' surprise," only 46 percent of health care professionals involved in clinical trials understood that a trial's purpose was to improve treatment for future patients. In explanation, the researchers pointed out that doctors are often torn: "On the one hand, they want to further research and improve treatment for the future. On the other hand, they are committed to helping the patients standing in front of them. But these two obligations sometimes conflict, leaving physician-investigators with a dilemma."[10]

Even if consent forms explained in one-syllable words in large type and plain language that the therapy offered might help the participant though that's not the point of it, desperate patients won't get that message: it's not the one we want to hear, it's not the one we can emotionally afford to hear, especially when the trial appears to be our last faint hope. A research oncologist working on an experimental vaccine for prostate and kidney cancer says, "We make it clear that there is a possibility of adverse effects. We tell them the benefit is probably to the next generation of patients. And yet we know these patients are clinging to the hope that this will have an impact on their tumour." How can they not?[11]

❧

Clinical trials in this country are usually co-operative projects undertaken by many players, including the drug industry, research granting councils, the medical community, an ethics review board and the federal government. Here's how the process is supposed to work: the sponsor, perhaps a pharmaceutical company or a research group, applies to Health Canada for permission to conduct a trial, submitting a protocol outlining its objectives, methodologies and admission criteria. The sponsor must also justify that a clinical trial is worth whatever potential risks the drug might have and that the patients will not be exposed to "undue risk." Health Canada, as well as an independent research ethics review board, for example, a hospital review board, reviews the application.

Once a trial is approved, "experienced clinical investigators within the medical community initiate the clinical study under the supervision of the ethics review board, and with the funding of the sponsor. Within the process of clinical trials, Health Canada regulates the science by ensuring that the clinical trial is designed properly, while the sponsor, investigators and research ethics boards oversee the operation of the clinical trials, ensuring that all protocols are being followed. It is the researcher's responsibility to maintain the protocols and gather the data."[12] And report the results honestly.

There are problems here though, at several levels.

Trials cost big bucks. However, public funding is shrinking and the manufacturers of the products being tested are paying for the research, throwing the door wide open for bias to creep in. The "cozy connections," as biologist and ecologist Rachel Carson called the relationship between industry and regulatory bodies, is shortening the length of arm supposedly maintained between the two. Trial results favouring a new therapy over a traditional one are more likely if the study is funded by the new therapy's manufacturer.[13] A University of Toronto analysis of 70 studies of a controversial heart drug found that 96 percent of the researchers who supported the drug had ties to the companies that manufactured it, and only 37 percent of those critical of the drug had such ties.[14]

The approvals process is collapsing under the weight of applications to conduct trials. So many are being submitted now (the number has doubled in the last couple of years) that research ethics boards and Health Canada are swamped. Approvals can become almost a rubber-stamp process.

Critics say that the inspection and oversight process is flawed, with scant oversight of the research ethics boards, a situation that can have dangerous repercussions for trial subjects. In a clinical trial of the drug

Iressa (gefitinib), 170 patients in a cohort of 10,000 died in Japan. In relation to this development, the drug's manufacturer claimed that it had informed the regulatory bodies in all countries where Iressa drug trials were being conducted. But somehow this information didn't make it through to the Canadian participants. The ultimate side effect— death—was not mentioned in the consent forms they signed. Only mild diarrhea was.[15] The consent forms have since been changed.

Health Canada describes its inspection and monitoring activities in relation to clinical trials:

5.1.2 Inspection activity:
- Sponsors, Qualified Investigators, Contract Research Organizations and Site Management Organizations will be inspected.
- Up to 2% of all Canadian clinical trial sites will be inspected each year. . . . This represents approximately 80 inspections per year and is based on information that there are approximately 4000 on-going clinical trials in Canada. The total number of inspections may vary depending on the time required for investigations.
- Two types of inspections will be performed:
    - inspection during clinical trials, and
    - inspection after the completion of clinical trials.[16]

The reality can be different. At the Children's Hospital of Eastern Ontario (CHEO), a cancer trial went ahead without Health Canada approval and a child died after mistakenly being given too high a dose of the drug Interleukin-2. Another boy in the trial survived an overdose of the drug but had a severe reaction, which was never reported to Health Canada, even though the law requires the clinical trial sponsor to report all such outcomes. The sponsor went ahead with the trial, and seven others like it across the country, without filing an application with Health Canada.[17] The Canadian representative for the trial's sponsor suggested that it was more important to offer the drug trials to the children than to meet Health Canada's requirements.

Lawyers say allowing unauthorized trials to continue discredits Canada's clinical trial system; bioethicists say such cases expose a weakness in Canada's clinical trial system.

Although the system is open to abuses and mistakes, oncologists must depend on this very system to help them help patients make decisions about their treatment. To look too closely at the cracks would mean they'd have to start questioning the entire structure. On the whole, it works. But it's frightening when it breaks down. Especially if your life depends in it.

In 1994, it was discovered that a Canadian doctor had been submitting false data on patients to ensure they met the strict eligibility criteria of the biggest breast cancer clinical trials program in history, the National Surgical Adjuvant Breast and Bowel Project (NSABBP), which guides the direction of standard breast cancer treatment. He had been doing this for 13 years. His transgressions came to the public's notice when a reporter broke the story; the regulatory authorities and the researchers running the trials knew what he'd been doing for at least three years before but had kept mum. The doctor had two defences for his actions—I guess if you didn't like his first one, you could choose his second, because they certainly offered two opposing takes: he said that the alterations he had made in up to 100 files were just "silly mistakes," and that he had altered files for the good of his patients, to ensure they had the best medical attention available. However, most oncologists will tell you that your quality of care is not affected if you are in a trial or not. Perhaps this doctor meant that if you are in a trial you are tracked more closely, because of the need to collect data for the study. In any event, it is unethical to entice patients into trials with such assurances. It's damaging to women who either don't fit the criteria of a protocol in trial or who choose not to participate in a trial, and it sets up expectations that might not be met for women who do. As well, one detail patients often miss is the (usually) one in three chance that they will be assigned to the standard arm of treatment, the treatment in current use that they'd be given even if they hadn't entered the trial.

Because of this doctor's actions—and not only his, as it was discovered in the ensuing audit that other doctors had been doing the same thing—all data in the trials involved were re-evaluated. It was subsequently announced that the alterations had made no difference to the study findings. All was well, we were told. But all was certainly not well: the biggest casualty of this episode was trust, which in the end is the true bedrock of medical treatment. Patients' trust in doctors, doctors' trust in researchers, the medical and scientific communities' faith in the clinical trial system, all were eroded. As one of the Canadian patients in the Iressa drug trial said, "You start mistrusting. And you start giving up hope. And as a cancer patient, all you've really got is hope."[18]

In 2001, 80,000 clinical trials were being conducted in the United States. Involving 20 million people as research subjects, they looked at everything from toothpaste to Taxol. In eight years, the number of anti-cancer drugs in trials has jumped from 124 to more than 400.[19] It is growing more and more difficult to find subjects for clinical trials, maybe because there are so many trials now, or maybe because of eroded trust. This shortage of subjects has led some pharmaceutical companies to hire marketing professionals to find patients.[20]

Doctors and researchers despair of this development. Shail Verma, an oncologist at the Ottawa Regional Cancer Centre, says by far the majority of women with breast cancer refuse to go into a clinical trial. "It baffles scientists today why there is this huge refusal rate," he says. "Part of it is a certain level of suspicion about the intention of the trial, the science of the trial, the toxicity of the trial, agreed, but there's also a proportion of thinking that says, I'll wait until someone else does this and then I'll accept it."[21]

When I asked Dr. Verma if he would go into a trial if he had cancer, he did not hide his ambiguous feelings: "I don't know. A family member refused to go into a trial. I told them you have to weigh the benefits and the risks. And in the end they refused. Humans behave differently in different circumstances. It's all very fine and dandy for me to pontificate about this but . . ."

Some doctors and scientists are not so sanguine about clinical trials when they face them from the prone position of the examining table, instead of from their customary vertical role. Dr. David Horrobin has been involved in medical research for decades; he has medical and doctorate degrees from Oxford University, has taught at several universities, edits two biomedical journals, founded a biotech company and is executive chairman of another, so you can believe him when he writes, "'I am thoroughly acquainted with the many important ethical and statistical issues that impinge on clinical trials.'"[22] Then he was diagnosed with mantle cell lymphoma, told that he had just six months to live and found himself in "a universe parallel to the one in which I had lived for 30 years."

That's when he discovered the divergence between expectations of patients and of scientists. Patients are looking for the best treatments in order to survive their own cancer; "the idea that altruism [volunteering to go into a trial to benefit future generations] is an important consideration for most patients with cancer is a figment of the ethicist's and statistician's imagination," Horrobin writes. Not to mention the imagination of my former ear doctor. "I believe that patients who are asked to volunteer for large trials in cancer . . . are being misled," he says. "Most such trials cannot be justified on ethical grounds." Horrobin also found to his dismay that "'in oncology, with few exceptions, effect sizes were very small.' In other words, few cancer treatments have a demonstrably big effect on the . . . disease."[23]

Oncologist Shail Verma would disagree: for instance, in relation to the clinical trial of dose-dense therapy, he says the results are really "exciting." "They show a 3 percent improvement—I don't know how people value 3 percent, how women value 3 percent. The study was over four years; statistics say, because of the size of the study [big], this is a significant difference. I value any improvement, even 1 percent with no increased toxicity. That's of value."

Maybe for the researcher, but for a woman with breast cancer, 3 percent seems pretty small. And how to ensure that you are among that 3 percent? No one knows yet how to do that.

Another contentious issue with clinical trials is that, because of the prohibitive cost, only large commercial enterprises can afford to put a drug through the trial system. In 1979, it cost on average US$54 million to develop and test a new drug; in 1991, it cost US$231 million. By 1998, the average cost was estimated to be between US$300 million and US$600 million,[24] and by 2001, it had risen even higher, to US$802 million per drug.[25]

The costs are high not only because it takes 10 to 15 years of exhaustive testing to get a drug to the marketplace but because, for every drug that gets there, there are thousands that don't. The cost of *that* research has to be absorbed into the price of the drug that is approved.

But what are the options? A look at medicine before the strictures and restraints of clinical trials is an encouragement to cling to the system, even with all its warts. In those days, when science got loose in the corridors of medicine, it killed patients at an alarming rate. Dr. Francis Moore, a renowned American surgeon whose experiments on patients laid the foundation for, among other things, organ transplants, heart-valve surgery and hormonal therapy against breast cancer, believed, for most of his life, that a doctor's responsibility was to employ "any effective means available" to cure patients. And if there weren't any? Then the doctor must come up with one: death was not acceptable. But "he did not hesitate to expose his patients to suffering and death if a new idea made scientific sense to him," writes Atul Gawande in *The New Yorker*.[26] According to his peculiar logic, Moore was killing people to save them; they just weren't the same people.

Confronted with the sure, usually swift and painful death of metastatic breast cancer patients in the mid-1950s, Moore began to look at the growing evidence that hormones somehow promoted the disease. Based on little more than a hunch, he and a colleague began removing the pituitary gland—a small nerve centre in the brain that controls everything from estrogen to human growth hormone—from breast cancer patients. "The operation would shut down their endocrine systems and thereby, Moore hoped, eliminate a major stimulus of cancer growth," writes Gawande.[27] This tremendously risky procedure unfortunately shut down many of the patients, too: some lost their sight, some their sense of smell, three had major strokes, seven developed seizures and one died. But one woman went into remission for 14 months, and a few others experienced a shrinking of their bone metastases. Spurred on by this apparent success—at least by scientific if not human standards—Moore continued experimenting and found that removing the ovaries and adrenal glands was less risky and as successful. Other physicians began to do similar work and the hunt was on to find a drug that could provide the same effect as these surgical approaches. These efforts laid the trail to tamoxifen and other hormonal therapies that are the standard treatments of today.

Even when his patients died because of his experiments, Moore persevered, never admitting to doubts about what he was doing until his first attempts at liver transplants in the early 1960s. Nine patients, nine horrific deaths. He never experimented with a major new therapy in human beings again. Yet, if that had always been his way, would we have hormone therapies today? Would we have organ transplants? Medical progress requires "a steady supply of the new and different, the bold, the shocking, even the outrageous";[28] it also requires compassion and care and honesty.

Critics of the clinical trial system think it could be improved if:

- trial proposals had to demonstrate in pre-clinical work that the "experimental" therapy compared favourably with the gold standard treatment;
- national standards were imposed for all drug trials;
- an effective monitoring system were imposed in relation to research ethics boards; and
- there were mandatory publishing of trial data.

So, here you are with another decision to make. How do you decide whether to go into a clinical trial? First, don't be rushed or bamboozled into a fast decision. When I was told that I was eligible for a trial, I was also told that I had to decide immediately because it was about to be closed to new participants. I rejected the trial, not so much on the basis of information but more on the basis of fear and anger—not the recommended foundations for decision making.

It's important to know what you are accepting or rejecting, and why, so ask a lot of questions:

- How long will the trial last? (That is, when will results about efficacy of the therapy being tested be available?)
- Where does the trial originate?
- What treatments will be used, and how?
- What is the main purpose of the trial?
- How is patient safety monitored?
- Are there any risks involved?
- What are the possible benefits?
- What are other treatments available besides the one being tested in the trial?
- Who is sponsoring the trial?
- Do I have to pay for any part of the trial?
- What happens if I am harmed by the trial?
- Can I opt out of the trial partway through?
- Can I opt to remain on this treatment, even after termination of the trial?[29]

Then follow your instincts. I am not being glib here; it really is the only way sometimes.

7

THE NEW REALITY: ALTERED PERSPECTIVES

Reality is the beginning not the end.

—Wallace Stevens, "An Ordinary Evening in New Haven"

FRIENDS, RELATIVES, COLLEAGUES respond to the news of your breast cancer in a variety of ways: the toughest ones to handle are the two extremes: the stark fear and the cheery kiss-off. There are some who respond to it as to a death announcement, their faces crumpling with pity and grief, thus confirming your own worst fears. Others greet your news with the blithe reassurance, "Oh, you'll be fine, there are such good treatments now that can cure cancer." The suggestion is that what you have is something slightly worse than a bad cold. The truth lies somewhere in between, and it is a fine line for you, let alone the people close to you, to understand and hang onto.

A brilliant piece of dialogue in the script for *Ladies in Waiting*, a research-based drama about breast cancer, says it all—the 10 things "survivors" don't want to hear:

Alice: You're so strong—such an inspiration to us all.
Naya:—Too much pressure.
Persephone: You can put it all behind you now.
Naya: Some can—but many of us can't. Too many post-treatment
  side effects.
Alice: I wouldn't worry about it. It's probably nothing.
Naya: That's what they said about the lump.
Persephone: Have you tried . . . ?
Naya: Either I have, or I don't want to hear about it.
Alice: Should you be eating, drinking, doing that?
Naya: Piss off.
Persephone: I have a friend who recently died of breast cancer.
Naya: Is this meant to cheer me up?
Alice: You should be grateful to be alive.
Naya: Oh puke!
Persephone: I know exactly how you feel.
Naya: Like hell.
Alice: We could all be hit by a bus tomorrow.
Persephone: You are one of the lucky ones.
Naya: Where's that bus when you need it!"[1]

My favourite is the "hit by a bus" line of solace. I'm not sure where
the comfort is in this traffic accident comparison: are you supposed to
be relieved that it was cancer and not a bus that hit you? That it could
be worse—that you could be dead immediately by bus rather than
dead slowly by cancer? Or is it a kind of existential observation on the
transience of security, the unpredictability of fate? I don't know, but
that line of compassion has always mystified me.

However it is expressed, though, the sympathy is heartfelt. First you
struggle through the reality of your disease and so do your friends and
family; then you struggle through treatment and so do, vicariously,
your friends and family. Then you wait for the good feelings to wash
over you and so do your friends and family. And the good feelings do

arrive, but not by themselves. There is the over-the-moon delight that it is finished—no more visits to the chemotherapy room, no more almost daily blood tests, no more lying under the glaring eye of the radiation machine, no more agendas driven by what day it is in the chemo cycle, no more days spent wondering if you are going to feel well enough to do anything or whether it will be another day you spend deep-sixed in chemo-induced nausea. You get your life back. And you are so glad, even if you feel lousy; you are so glad, even if you find yourself squeezed by fear or fogged in a depression that feels as if it will never lift.

One woman said that when she finished treatment, she promptly had a panic attack. Another said it was like falling off a conveyor belt. For most of us, these feelings are unexpected, inexplicable, threading the elation with a low-level dread that grips you in a limbo of waiting. You've survived this bout, but you find that you are now waiting for the next one. You keep thinking that this is just Round One.

These reactions surprise us and often exasperate friends and family, and even our physicians. "I feel like doctors think that I complain too much, like I should [just] be happy that I am alive," one woman commented, ". . . I am alive, but I still have needs and issues that are important."[2]

"Let it go," a friend might say, with the best intentions. "Get on with your life. I know lots of women who don't dwell on their cancer; they just put it behind them." And lots of women do. They move on, parking their breast cancer in the past, as if it never happened. But many can't shake off the tentacles of the disease, or at least the fear it has instilled.

There is more than a suggestion that you are just being a wimp, that you are hanging onto the fear to get more attention. You are expected to get back to normal, and you really want to, but the old normal has vanished. For some lucky ones, it's vanished only temporarily, but for others, it's gone for good, as it has for the characters in *Ladies in Waiting:*

Persephone: Excuse me. Does the bus to Normal stop here?
Naya: So they say.
Persephone: Have you been waiting long?
Alice: Years.
Persephone: So the bus doesn't come very often?
Naya: I haven't seen it yet.[3]

Breast cancer is a new reality. Many of us must make personal and poignant adjustments to travel within it; some move into its public arena, which, when viewed up close, can require adjustments at another level. Here, you are faced with the political issues that, as long as breast cancer was nothing more than a free-floating fear out there, back in your old reality, would have passed you by.

RECALIBRATING NORMAL

Remember that message you'd sometimes get on TV? "The interference you are experiencing is temporary. Please do not adjust your set." With breast cancer, it's the opposite. The interference for most is not temporary. And you do need to adjust your set—for "set" read your sense of normal—and so does everyone around you.

You must adapt to the loss of your old self in one way or another, to the loss of the you who blithely banged along down the days among the fixtures of life you assumed were immutable. The thing is, they are, you aren't. And that's a shock. Fitting the changed you into your old life often doesn't work. The fit isn't there any more.

Breast cancer, for most women, alters. There are the obvious physical alterations. On the eve of surgery—whether for a lumpectomy or full mastectomy—it is truly shocking to realize that this body you've had all your life, for better or worse, in 12 hours will be forever *altered*. And through the various stages of treatment it continues to be altered— it may be that more flesh is carved off or out, or that chemotherapy forever plants in your unconscious a Pavlovian response to, say, the sight of needles, or a white coat and stethoscope, unleashing a surge of nausea, not imagined but an altered neurological reality.

❦

A few months after Nicole had her first mastectomy, she elected to have a second. It was only partly prophylactic. She wanted to give the cancer one less foothold, but there was another reason. She hated the asymmetry. It weighed on her both literally and figuratively. She wore a prosthesis for a while but it was a nuisance, so she abandoned it. She went to see a surgeon about reconstruction but came away thinking, "Why bother, it's no big deal." But the lack of balance was. It was not natural. It was abnormal. By deciding to have her second breast amputated, Nicole regained the symmetry she missed. And it was the right decision for her. She swam, she skied, she hiked, she moved through her old space with a new balance—she had adjusted her standards of normal to be able to function in her new world.

Mary Trafford had a different symmetry to achieve. Her first huge adjustment to living in the kingdom of the ill came in 1964. She was 11 years old, a tall, skinny, active kid with a sore knee. She ignored the pain for a while—doesn't every kid get a sore knee some time or other, especially a kid like Mary who was always on the move, who never stopped running, playing and riding? "I was taken to the doctor eventually and went from a casual medical appointment to—boom—right into the Montreal General Hospital for three months," she remembers. "At the time, I was never actually told what I had."[4]

It was osteogenic sarcoma of the right femur—the same cancer Terry Fox had—a very aggressive cancer with a high rate of recurrence. The five-year survival prognosis at the time Mary was diagnosed was 4 percent. Her doctor took an unorthodox approach to treatment. "The normal approach then would have been immediate amputation and chemotherapy, but he really wanted to save the leg so he did radiation therapy . . . and some form of chemotherapy that was injected directly into the artery [of the leg]."

Mary recovered, but her leg didn't. "There was a lot of radiation damage and complications, and even though I had the leg, it was not really functional. I went for about three years, until the spring of 1967, when it was decided that it had to be amputated after all. I had to go to New York City because no one in this area could do the kind of surgery that was needed, a hemipelvectomy . . . a rare type of amputation; usually you only see it from traumatic injury, motorcycle accidents, or for cancer of the pelvis."

The decision to amputate wasn't made because the cancer had come back, Mary says. "Whatever the problem was with the leg, it seemed as if it was draining the health out of me. I was weak, I had no appetite, my mobility was poor, I was down to 91 pounds. . . . Once I had had the amputation and got over the post-surgery trauma, I remember waking up in my room in the New York University hospital with an appetite, which I hadn't had for what seemed like time immemorial. My cousin came in with cold homemade roast chicken and I basically devoured it. I started eating then and I've never stopped," she laughs. "Then I was just healthy—I know there were terrible concerns, I know my family doctor in Manotick expected me to drop dead any day."

The delay of three years in amputating her leg gave Mary an adjustment period that she feels protected her from the worst of the shock of such a horrific development. By the time it became evident that the leg had to go, Mary was ready, because it had become a burden—"this stupid leg," she called it. It was preventing her from doing what she loved best—horseback riding; it was preventing her from adjusting and moving on.

Mary had accepted that the "interference" caused by her cancer was not temporary. And she made the adjustments necessary to create for herself a new normal, a life in which she could ride her horse. That was what mattered. "I remember when the doctor told me that I'd have to lose the leg, I asked him if I would still be able to ride after the surgery, and I'm sure he didn't have a clue, I'm sure of it, but he said yes without even hesitating. It was a good thing that he said that, because as far as I was concerned, it was, fine, then let's get on with it, because basically for three years I had been pretty much incapacitated by this stupid leg. Once I got home and was well again, I got my own horse—horses were the normalizing thing for me."

Mary's "normal" took another jolt in 1998 when cancer struck again, this time in her breast. It was DCIS. She elected for a mastectomy. Now the worry was, aside from everything else, how was she going to use her crutches, which she has had since she was 14. (A leg prosthesis had never been an option for her because of the extent of the surgery.) Somehow, this latest assault to her body had to be accommodated to the first one; adjustments had to be made. Mary is a strong, independent woman; so much so, she chose to leave the hospital the same day as her surgery: "Being the stubborn mule that I am, I went home, which was really stupid for a lot of reasons. For one, [the surgeon] forbade me from using my crutches . . . and Sue [Mary's partner] had to figure out how she was going to get me home. She rushed out and rented me a wheelchair, and even though I insisted I could get to the washroom, she rented a commode which I was furious about. . . . After a week or so I was up and about and I could use my crutches and it didn't hurt . . . well, not really."

Mary laughs about her struggle to tame the initial breast prosthesis, the "puffball," as she calls it. "They have this 'puffball room' at the Canadian Cancer Society office, full of cardboard boxes of fabric boobs . . . nobody was there, it was like, 'There's the room, help yourself.' So you go in and dig around in the boxes and pull out one, and say, Is this the right size? Well, no, how about this one? . . . They are very, very light, so light they can go from being a breast to a shoulder pad in no time!" The one she has now is "a kind of blended combination, part filled with silicone and part with talcum powder to give it the right weight."

Mary's way of recalibrating "normal" was to make her body even stronger to compensate for the missing parts. She joined the breast cancer dragon-boat team. "Within a month, I started exercising with a videotape, building strength more than anything—I knew Nicole was on the team, so it became my goal." She pauses for a moment, then adds, "Of course, [I didn't join the team] that same summer. I joined the next year."

As for asymmetry? That was the least of her worries. "I did consult with a breast reconstruction surgeon, but I'm not even a candidate. The asymmetry doesn't bother me; I mean, I'm used to it," she laughs, gesturing at where her leg used to be. And Sue is not bothered either. "Maybe she likes the variety," Mary says. "And we both felt, why would you put yourself through that surgery?"

When reconstruction is an option, more and more women are opting for it as one of the ways to achieve a renewed sense of normal. Even though there have been big advances in reconstruction surgery, it remains a major undertaking, either done with implants or requiring extensive surgery to other parts of the body—the abdomen, buttocks, back or thighs—to gather up the fat and flesh to build new breasts. The reconstructed breasts do not have nerve endings in the tissue; they might feel good to the feeler, but there's no sensation for the "feelee." And although technology and procedures in this area are improving, it's still important to find a plastic surgeon who has lots of experience in breast reconstruction. Mistakes can be undone, but as one woman said, it is "massive amounts of no fun." She was talking about the whole experience of breast cancer in general, the replacement of leaking implants in particular.

Barb Crooks was diagnosed in 1990 and had a mastectomy followed by chemotherapy, followed by a second prophylactic mastectomy. "[At first,] I didn't mind my flat chest at all. I was like a young boy," Barb says. "And it didn't trouble John [her husband] either. Often I wouldn't even bother wearing Wanda and Wilma," the names she had given her two prostheses.[5]

However, six years after her second mastectomy, Barb decided to have a full bilateral reconstruction. It took her a long time to find the right surgeon, and the courage, to do it. "I kept booking and then cancelling the surgery," Barb says. Finally, she went to Toronto for a "tram flap" procedure. "This is when they split the abdominal muscles and slide stomach fat up under the skin to form the breasts. It's major surgery." Barb and her husband were told that the procedure would take about five hours. "John was in the waiting room and saw the surgeon coming down the hall after less than two hours. 'Oh, my God, she's died,' was his first thought. I hadn't," she says dryly. But reconstruction surgery was being done so frequently by then that the surgeon had a team trained in the specific skills needed, allowing the operation to go much faster. Barb later took the final step and had nipples tattooed onto her new breasts. She says that they need to be redone about every six months.

Barb tells of a friend who eventually adjusted to her new normal in a very decisive way. In a sense, breast cancer allowed her to make a major decision that she realized was long overdue. She'd had a mastectomy 11 years before, and after she saw Barb's reconstructed breasts, "my beautiful new boobs," Barb says with pride, "she was so impressed, she said, 'I'm going to do that, too.'"

After she had healed from the reconstructive surgery, she bought a sexy nightgown—for years she had been sleeping in old T-shirts. When her husband saw it, he was less than supportive. "What's *this* all about?" he sneered.

Something snapped. "Out," she ordered. "Get out." This, after 26 years of marriage. "She hadn't known until she said the words, that this was how she felt," Barb says. Her new breasts had given her a new self-confidence, had empowered her into regaining herself and ditching a husband with whom she had been miserable for years.

⁓

Helen Humphreys, in her novel *The Lost Garden,* describes what happens in wartime to people forced, physically and figuratively, out of their lives, not through illness or death but through dislocation. "I realize we haven't left our lives. They have left us. The known things in them. The structure of our days . . . We have been abandoned by the very facts of ourselves, by the soft weight of the old world."[6] With breast cancer, with any disease that may be terminal, it is exactly the opposite. Our bodies, our thoughts change—the "soft weight" of the old world doesn't. Take dill pickles, for instance.

In the research-based drama about women with metastatic breast cancer *Handle with Care,* one of the characters, Jan, has just learned that she has to have more treatment and worries that she won't be able to finish making her pickles. She's already bought the cucumbers and dill; now they'll be wasted. She turns to the audience and asks, "Who needs seventy-eight jars of homemade pickles?" She's not asking who will take them off her hands. It's a philosophical question, one of life's conundrums, this pickle question. The answer is, of course, *no one* needs 78 jars of pickles, at least not in the vinegary, garlicky reality of a green condiment lurking on your preserve shelves; but as metaphor, many of us need those pickles desperately. Jan, in the play, explains their importance: "I've established myself as the best dill pickle maker in my family. It's a title I bear proudly and work hard to maintain."[7] It's part of who she is, part of her sense of self, a self from her old world that she does not want to lose in the new one.

She enlists a friend to do the heavy work, which is to lug the pickles to the cellar and run them through the washing machine on the cold-water, gentle-wash cycle. What? No way. They'd come out relish, wouldn't they? Apparently only if you spin them dry.

I nearly jumped out of my skin when I heard this piece of dialogue. *I'd* bought cucumbers—a bushel of them—and, before I had a chance to do anything with them, I was told I had breast cancer. There is a certain imperative about a bushel of pickling cucumbers, sitting in your kitchen, each day threatening to soften, bruise, rot and turn to slime. It takes enormous strength of will, which I did not have, to ignore their ominous, brooding presence. Despite the apparent death sentence I'd just been handed, they still occupied space in my reeling brain. I worried about getting those damn pickles finished. Your world has just ended, but it hasn't. The pickles are waiting. All the little things, the routines, the tasks and duties, all the stuff that keeps us anchored in our lives does not necessarily go away. The tough part is that in a sense *we* have gone away. Even breast cancer could not knock Jan out of her autumn routine. It was part of who she was, it was normalcy. Who knew where she'd be in six weeks when the pickles were ready. I didn't think about that either, at first. All I knew was that it was of utmost importance not to let those cucumbers rot. I didn't know then about the washing machine trick (which, by the way, works), so I enlisted my family to scrub, prick and pack, and the brine grew saltier with my secret tears as I faced the seeming certainty that I wouldn't be around the next autumn to do this task again. Maybe not even in six weeks, to eat them. That was 20 years ago, and every year when I make pickles, it is an unspoken celebration; it is my green metaphor for yearly survival.

WHEN BAD GETS WORSE

There are less whimsical weights from the old world, hard imperatives that do not miraculously disappear just because you suddenly have to deal with harder ones. They come with you like baggage not wanted on the voyage and require even more adjustment and accommodation in the land of the ill. These are the social determinants—poverty, age, sexual preference, race, language, geographical location—that can rule a woman's world at the best of times, but when the best gets bad, these can make things so much worse. In the corridors of cancer, or any illness, their impact can tip the balance between getting well or getting sicker.[8]

It's bad enough to be elderly and frail, worse to get breast cancer and be shuffled to the bottom of the health care priority list because of your age. It's bad enough for lesbians to have to deal with social prejudice, worse to get breast cancer and have that prejudice become a barrier to optimum health care. It's bad enough to be poor, worse to get breast cancer and not be able to afford it.

Lisette Guérette, a social worker at the Dr. Léon Richard Oncology Centre in Moncton, sees the direct impact of money—specifically, the lack of it—every day on women's health: "I've seen people refusing to take medication because of the cost, drugs that could be very expensive and they don't have that kind of money, even with insurance."[9] These are drugs that could save or at least extend their lives. Or they might forgo anti-nausea drugs while on chemotherapy because they can't afford them. The cost of the chemo drugs is covered because they are administered within the hospital, but the anti-nausea drugs are not. Lisette says, "Some cost as much as $25 a pill; if you have to take five a day, that's $125 a day, and this is outside the hospital—this is where the expense lies. You have to be admitted to the hospital to have your medication covered. If you are out [of hospital], you are out . . . of luck."

The TV documentary on breast cancer *Reasons for Hope* features three white, middle-class women with supportive husbands, lovely houses and, apparently, a reasonable amount of money.[10] Their lives may reflect those of many women, but not the reality for many others. This is not to downplay their experience, nor to suggest that it is not harrowing, difficult and frightening; it is. But women who must wrestle with so many other issues are often overlooked in the media and fundraising hoopla around the disease, which makes adjusting to their new normal a lonely exercise.

In this documentary, one of the women is filmed in a garden, presumably at her home, playing with her son and dog. The expanse of grass is rich and manicured; shrubs and flowers border it in an orderly fashion. She talks about the importance of getting your priorities right when you have breast cancer. She says that she didn't work too much any more and instead put her family first; that money wasn't her top priority, although she knew that for lots of people it was. It shouldn't be, she says, because you never know what is going to happen to you and having lots of money isn't going to help you.

In her context, this statement made sense. I think she means, don't focus on making *more* money a priority. In the context of a woman who does not have money, who does not have the choice of not making it top priority, this advice is hard to take. It certainly doesn't reflect the experience of a young woman Lisette Guérette spoke of who has two kids, a husband on employment insurance and cancer and can come nowhere near being able to afford the $3,000 shortfall between what her insurance covers and what she'd have to pay herself for elements of her treatment. It doesn't reflect the woman who hasn't enough money for bus fare to get to the hospital for treatment, or to pay for lunch in the hospital cafeteria while she waits between appointments. Or the woman who has to reject drugs she needs because she hasn't got a medical plan to cover the costs. Or the woman who is still struggling six years later to pay off the debts incurred by her first round of treatment. Or the woman who is a single parent, who does not have help at home during her treatments, who can't afford a babysitter on hospital appointment days, who can hardly see to the end of the day, let alone the end of the long dark tunnel that has become her life.

People who have money can afford the economic cost of having breast cancer, and "people who have no money, they are okay; they go to the welfare office and they are eligible for assistance," says Lisette. But even in Canada, with our universal medical system, to afford the luxury of getting sick, you either have to be broke or rich; there seems to be no in-between.

Lisette says that many breast cancer patients turn to the Canadian Cancer Society for financial help and are astonished and angry when it is not forthcoming. "[They] don't understand that the CCS can't help them directly. They are not happy with that. They say, 'Why can't they help me? I gave money to the cancer society all my life. . . . Now I have cancer, the cancer society should help me.'"

The Canadian Cancer Society (CCS) has been this country's public face of cancer for decades, especially in small communities. Eleanor Nielson, director of Patient Services and Public Education at the national office until her retirement in 2003, points out that the CCS is primarily a fundraising organization for the National Cancer Institute of Canada; hence, most of the dollars go to research and not to individuals in need. The Society does have two specific service programs. Reach to Recovery, probably its best-known direct service, is a one-to-one peer support program in which volunteers who have had cancer visit newly diagnosed patients to provide moral support. Cancer Connection is a telephone linkage program to match people with the same cancers, designed most specifically for people living in rural areas who might not be able to find someone in their community with a shared experience.

Women living in the country or a small town a distance from the treatment centre, usually in a large urban centre, face other worries— the time and expense of travelling, and, in some instances, the cost of accommodation during treatment. Some treatment centres have residential facilities, but often as not, women must make their own arrangements, which can be expensive. Or they might have to land in on a friend or relative, which brings with it its own stresses. The biggest stress, of course, is being away from their own home and family at a time when they need both most. Some women commute, but this can be both exhausting and time-consuming. For women who can't drive, this means finding someone who can, regularly.

Madeleine H. had to drive to a treatment centre for radiation therapy from her home more than three hours away. When I asked her how she felt about the radiation, she replied, "You know the biggest hassle of my treatment? It's getting here for it."[11] For another woman, that hassle was just too much to deal with, at least in winter. She refused to go to the centre for treatment until spring because of the icy roads. She was to have started treatment in December.

One young woman was a three-hour drive from where she was to have radiation treatment. It was September, she had three children starting back at school and although she was urged to stay at the residential cancer lodge during the week, she refused, choosing to do a seven-hour-a-day commute. "I have to be home when my kids come home from school." The radiation unit did its best to have her treatment scheduled for the morning so that she could leave home at the same time as her children, then get back just before they got home from school. She did this for 25 days.

Commitments and priorities don't go away when you get breast cancer. You just need to make even greater adjustments in your new life to accommodate them.

Being younger or older than the statistical average age of women who get breast cancer has an impact too. Many young women with breast cancer (defined as under age 45 at time of diagnosis) find that in their new world, "nothing fits." They aren't talking about clothes. "Ill-fitting" experiences range from diagnosis, throughout treatment and at follow-up.[12] Many say that although there is lots of information out there, most of it is irrelevant to their specific needs or what they need is missing altogether. They say it is difficult to find out about the effects of adjuvant therapies on fertility, or about the signs and side effects of menopause brought on by treatment; they want but can't get good advice on how to talk about their cancer in new relationships, how to relate to themselves sexually following treatment and how to talk to their children about their cancer.

Misconceptions about young women and breast cancer make their lives even harder. They range from "young women don't get breast cancer" to "young women shouldn't get breast cancer, and if they do, it is their own fault for making bad lifestyle choices" to "young women all die of breast cancer because they always get the most virulent kind." All wrong, but still out there. One woman said that she became infertile as a result of treatment she had in her late 20s. Twelve years later, she wanted to adopt a baby but was not approved; the fact that she had had breast cancer made her an "unfit" mother, even though she has been cancer-free ever since.[13]

Following her diagnosis and treatment, 31-year-old Carole LeBlanc joined the Reach to Recovery program to help other young women in her same plight. "They try to match me with young people . . . in the last year, I've seen more young women than ever before. . . . I leave my phone number and say to call if they want. Some do, some don't. People cope in different ways. One woman couldn't even look at herself for a month, she was taking showers with her shirt on."[14]

One young woman summed it up: "When you are young and you get a cancer diagnosis I believe it changes the entire trajectory of your life . . . I don't think it happens as much with an older person because they've had more of the foundations of their life."[15]

Older women have other issues to face. When a woman over, say, 75 gets breast cancer, she might not be offered the option of adjuvant therapy following a mastectomy or lumpectomy on the grounds that she doesn't have that much longer to live anyway. "It's not any easier for a seventy-four-year-old woman to die of breast cancer than it is for a thirty-three-year-old. It's unjust to say that because you're seventy-four you should just grin and bear it," says a character in the research-based drama about women with breast cancer, *Handle with Care*.[16]

Mary Trafford's mother had two mastectomies, and Mary says of the scars, "One was vertical and one was horizontal, and I always thought it was poorly done surgery, that the surgeon hadn't cared what it looked like. [My mother] claimed she didn't care either, but she did. After that surgery, she really deteriorated psychologically."

This is also the age group most likely to put their own needs second, third, fourth down the list. A mother might put off hip replacement surgery, even though she is in agony, because she is needed to take care of a new grandchild. My mother put off telling us about a lump that had been found in her breast and delayed the biopsy until after Christmas because she didn't want to ruin our holiday. The biopsy was positive, and a mastectomy was done right away, while she was still under anaesthesia, a practice that has been largely discontinued. When she came to, heavily bandaged and groggy, she had no idea what had been done and the nurses couldn't tell her. Only the doctor can tell you that, they said. The catch was, the doctor had left for the weekend. It took my sister and me all day to track him down. We finally caught up with him at home, and he wasn't pleased. No need to get hysterical, he said. (By then, we were ready to rip his head off.) "Your mother is 72, you know. Is it such a big deal to lose a breast at her age?"

That was 30 years ago. Times should have changed. And they have, but not enough. There is still a tendency in Western society in general to assume that the needs of older women are not as important as those of younger women. Many accept this relegation to second-class citizenship, an attitude that can leave them vulnerable to suggestions that they aren't or shouldn't be as important as others in the cancer care system. What was a social bias in their old universe can become a life and death issue in their new one.

Lesbians face even more blatant discrimination. One woman commented that it was like "coming out" two times: first to acknowledge that she was lesbian, second to acknowledge that she had breast cancer.[17] "I am marked twice," she said. You'd think that breast cancer would be the great equalizer, wiping out all the pettiness of the old world, focusing everyone's energies on one goal—send this disease away. It doesn't seem to work that way. Sadly, stigmas are still alive and well and do not seem to stop at the border.

It is not clear whether lesbians are at increased risk for breast cancer. In the early 1990s, a US National Cancer Institute researcher said a new study showed that lesbians had a one-in-three lifetime risk of developing breast cancer. Panic. Turned out this was wrong, but damage had been done. The researcher hadn't looked at the data measuring the actual incidence of breast cancer among lesbians . . . because there was none. So she had compared known risk factors for breast cancer and looked to see whether they occurred more often in the lesbian population. They did. But that finding did not translate into a "breast cancer epidemic" ripping through the lesbian population, as was being claimed. Further research indicated that breast cancer rates are about 1 percent higher among lesbians, nothing close to the earlier estimates. "In other words, if 10 straight women out of 100 were likely to get breast cancer during their lifetime, the number would be 11 out of 100 for lesbians." Two factors might explain this slightly higher risk: fewer lesbians have children, hence are exposed longer to hormonal activity, and early detection is less likely because many lesbians feel isolated from traditional treatment and support systems and fear the disdain they may encounter from the medical establishment.[18]

The discrimination lesbians often face from their doctors is either a lack of understanding of particular issues they face or a studied denial of their situation. One woman reported the frustration she felt when her surgeon said to her, "'If breasts are important to you and your husband we can always do implants,' and he left. And I remember sitting there thinking, he forgot who I was. And I just thought, 'Oh, my God, I'm never going back to see that guy ever again.' Yet I have to go back—he's my only option in the city where I live. So I haven't done any follow-up. . . ."[19]

Another said that what she found more difficult than anything was "fighting the system on stupid little issues like, 'Could you be pregnant?' I don't know how many times I got asked that question. It's like, 'No, I'm a lesbian, and I've been in a committed relationship for the last nine years, there's no possible way that I could be pregnant.' 'We don't believe you; pee in the cup.' I often want to walk away sometimes when I have those battles."[20]

Just as for older women, such attitudes become tougher to handle in the world of the ill, because they can seriously jeopardize access to good health care.

THE PUBLIC—AND POLITICAL—LANDSCAPE

In your old world, when breast cancer was something other people got, your awareness of the disease might have been restricted to a free-floating fear each time you heard about another risk factor to avoid. You can't help but hear about it in October, when the whole month turns pink with the awareness and fundraising campaigns. When you have the disease, it has a different hue. That's when you discover that the world of breast cancer goes beyond the disease itself, a confusing mix of players and issues and competing interests. Groups that range from grassroots organizations to government agencies all strive toward the same goal but they don't always agree on how to achieve it.

In Canada, breast cancer officially "came out" in 1993 with the National Forum, at which a quarter of the 650 delegates were survivors and their families. "This once-silent constituency fused real life experience to theoretical debate," says Sharon Batt, a prominent writer and activist in the breast cancer community.[21] Before then, a hush shrouded cancer in mystery and shame. It is still referred to by many as "the big C," as if naming it might unleash its full menace. Like Valdemort, the evil wizard in the Harry Potter books, whose name could not be uttered aloud for fear of attracting his wicked attention, cancer was the disease "that must not be named." Breast cancer especially was taboo: "Something about the conjuncture of 'breast,' signifying sexuality and nurturance, and that other word, suggesting the claws of a devouring crustacean, spooked almost everyone."[22]

In many places and in many countries, the social stigma of breast cancer still holds women in a grip of silence; they would rather die than tell. For example, in India, many women consider that breast cancer is punishment for sins of a previous life, so are ashamed to tell anyone of their disease. In Zambia, many women believe that cancer is caused by witchcraft and are afraid to admit to the disease. In some Muslim countries, women can't make any decisions about their health; only their husbands or male members of their family do that, so many stay silent. There are rumblings in all these countries now, grassroots activities by and for women, to bring breast cancer out into the light where there is hope of treating and containing it. Left in secret and darkness, it will continue its inexorable killing. This is one battle, at least in North America, that we seem close to winning.[23]

It is rare now to hear of women who have gone to their grave with their secret of breast cancer intact. Women certainly still ignore early warning signs, but through fear rather than shame. The public awareness campaigns of the last couple of decades deserve credit for bringing the disease out of the closet. So do the lobby groups and advocacy groups determined to move the fight against breast cancer to centre stage, both at the government and community levels.

Such developments have influenced attitudes to do with other cancers: prostate cancer is now getting more public attention; men are speaking out; support groups are springing up and credit is given to the example set by what women have done in relation to breast cancer.

In the last 15 years, the public world of breast cancer has exploded with activity and organizations, all born out of the energy and anger and determination of women—as well as that of their families, friends and doctors—who have been touched by the disease. The Canadian Breast Cancer Network was created in 1994 to be "the national voice of breast cancer survivors." It now has 13 subsites across Canada, provides information and resources, works in advocacy and tries to eliminate duplication of services. This is a challenge because of the growing galaxy of players in the breast cancer community. Willow Breast Cancer Support and Resource Services (now called Willow Breast Cancer Support Canada) was launched that same year, survivor-driven and focusing specifically on two clearly identified needs: women with breast cancer wanted to talk to breast cancer survivors for support, and they wanted information tailored to their own situation. The Breast Cancer Support Network for Ontario, which integrated with Willow in 1997, helps women who want to start and facilitate community-based self-help groups, of which there are literally hundreds now across Canada. The Canadian Breast Cancer Foundation is the largest charitable organization in Canada that is dedicated to supporting the advance-ment of breast cancer research and education. With a national office and four regional chapters, it has allocated over $18 million in project grants. There are also several Breast Cancer Actions—Montreal, Ottawa, Kingston, Nova Scotia, Saskatchewan and Manitoba. The aim of these volunteer, survivor-led organizations is to educate and support people with breast cancer, as well as the community at large.

Added to the mix are the charitable foundations of hospitals, women's health coalitions, conference organizers and ad-hoc groups focused on single issues. Government agencies at the federal and provincial levels also have fingers in the pie, as do large corporations that have adopted breast cancer as their charity of choice. Such a disparate fellowship is bound to contain some uneasy bedfellows. For a newcomer to this world, the very number of organizations, as well as the occasional dust-ups, can be daunting. It's hard when you encounter rifts that gobble up valuable energy of women who do not have any energy to spare, and petty turf wars that sometimes obscure the main battle.

"I am a breast cancer survivor, yes," one woman told me at a fund-raiser, "but probably even more important," and her voice dropped to a conspiratorial whisper, "I am a breast cancer *organization* survivor." Followed by a great gust of laughter.

Breast cancer has mobilized women from every walk of life, but it hasn't necessarily unified them. It would be naïve to expect so, but I think lots of us did. A few years ago I wrote a feature report on breast cancer for a national magazine in which I quoted two women prominent in the movement. Their words happened to be in the same paragraph but on unrelated subjects. When the article appeared, one of the women let me know she was upset about the juxtaposition. The two women were at such loggerheads that she didn't even want her name to appear on the same page. They had started out as colleagues, fighting on the same side, struggling with the same issues. Yet a year later, they weren't speaking to each other. Within months, their common enemy, breast cancer, had killed one of them. Death has a way of putting things into perspective, but sometimes even it gets lost sight of in the skirmishes.

Many feel that death has been demoted to a bit player, shrouded in pink and tucked out of sight in what has become a veritable industry of awareness, a host of corporate-sponsored events to raise money and profile. "It's the breast cancer bandwagon," Sharon Batt says, "a horrible bandwagon, all these runs, and mugs and ribbons and bears . . .

it's become commodified. . . . The issue has been taken up by corporate entities for marketing, which is definitely a minus."[24]

One of the most divisive debates is about breast cancer as big business. "They're good girls and boys. Racing for the cure. Crying for the cameras. Sharing their pain. Wearing that crown of thorns like a halo. Nice folks. And aren't they 'better people' for just having 'survived' breast cancer?" This is the lead sentence in an article entitled "Breast Cancer Money-Go-Round"[25] that goes on to say that, no, we're not better people, we're suckers, conned by a clever marketing strategy. The anger boils from this article like acid. And it burns. Now, not only do you have to feel guilty about getting breast cancer because you did the wrong things, and guilty for dying from breast cancer because you did the wrong things, but now you have to feel guilty about *surviving* breast cancer because you are doing the wrong things. Enough, already.

The argument is that big business has co-opted breast cancer, not as a charity or social issue but as a marketing tool. One aspect of this development is "pharma funding," a particularly divisive issue, creating angst and dissension among many grassroots organizations in the breast cancer community. Some feel that by accepting money from a pharmaceutical company the organization loses its credibility as an independent—and trustworthy—entity. And the pharmaceutical company has gained a shill. Sharon Batt calls such organizations "astro-turf" groups, fake actors in the grassroots movement. Others disagree, saying such arrangements with big business are partnerships that allow the smaller organizations the financial wherewithal to do good work and provide needed services that otherwise wouldn't happen.

More and more businesses are tying their corporate identities to good causes, and "breast cancer has become the queen of all good causes."[26] It generates a staggering array of company tie-ins. You can buy recipe books for the cure and then cook for the cure with a pink KitchenAid mixer, golf for the cure with golf balls stamped with the ubiquitous pink ribbon; you can run, walk, bike for the cure (CIBC and Avon), clean for the cure (Eureka vacuum cleaners), charge for the cure (American Express); you can kiss breast cancer goodbye (Avon), you can target the cure (high-fashion T-shirts with a bull's eye logo (at the high-end store), kiss for the cure again (Revlon), wear a pink trench-coat for the cure (Burberry), accessorize for the cure with any number of pins and scarves, and you could stock a forest with all the teddy bears raising money for the cause.

So is this bad? The answer seems to be both a definite yes and no. All this activity raises awareness, which beats secrecy and stigma, as Barbara Ehrenreich, a writer who bubbles with anger at the world of pink kitsch she found herself in after getting breast cancer, says, "But I can't help noticing that the existential space in which a friend has earnestly advised me to 'confront [my] mortality' bears a striking resemblance to a mall."[27] Where mortality is not on display. However, some feel that the very success of these awareness campaigns could end up hurting the cause and may be responsible for their own demise. You sense it already. Overkill. Burnout. Some journalists have had it with the topic; so "last year" they say. We wish. The media saturation in October each year can lead women to believe that it isn't *if* they get breast cancer, it's *when* they get breast cancer, as if the disease is one of the stages in the ordinary progression of life, like menopause. The difficulty is that breast cancer the issue isn't something that you get too caught up in—until you get caught up in breast cancer the disease. "When you or a family member or friend gets hit, that's when it really gets your attention, and that kind of interest is not going to go away as long as women are being diagnosed in such large numbers."[28]

All this activity raises money, although some say more for the companies than for the cause. A corporate manager involved in a high-profile breast cancer campaign points out that when you're spending from your marketing budget and not your philanthropy budget, you look for a return on that investment. There is a counter-argument here, cynical or practical, your choice. These companies are going to be involved in some cause, even if only because they know it is good for their profile: customers are attracted to the image of a good corporate citizen and will seek out its products. So, is it not better for the breast cancer community to reap some of that financial benefit? Is it not better to take the money, put it to good use, and at the same time acknowledge that philanthropy and profit are uneasy bedfellows?

No, say many activists. They see such corporate involvement as exploitation, making profits on the backs of ill women. They see it as nothing short of a hijacking. They claim these campaigns trivialize the disease, "pinkwashing" its real nature. "Breast cancer is anything but childlike; it is so not about teddy bears and that cutesy girly stuff."[29] They object to the exclusive focus on finding a cure, which comes packaged with the subliminal message that that cure is some kind of drug and is coming to a hospital near you.

Many feel that we should be running for the cause not the cure, but this isn't happening because it would send us on a route that could involve going up against the very companies that are sponsoring the campaigns. It is often pointed out, for example, that breast cancer awareness month (October) was co-created several years ago by AstraZeneca, a pharmaceutical company whose parent company manufactures pesticides and which makes tamoxifen, the drug that oncologist Shail Verma says, with understatement, everyone is getting "cranky" about, especially as chemoprevention. It's time to move past awareness, activists say, and toward "meaningful action," such as lobbying governments for systemic change. These campaigns, they claim, siphon the finite energy of women, which could be better used in action at the social and political levels.

These are all intellectually convincing arguments, but when I tried to explain them to Erin, one of my daughters-in-law, I was brought up short when she asked, "Does that mean we shouldn't go into the run for the cure?" She and her mother, and both my sons, have run in the CIBC-sponsored event each October, and this meant so much to me. And my other daughter-in-law, Erinn, and I completed the Princess Margaret Hospital Weekend to End Breast Cancer 60 km walk in September 2007. Such participation had nothing to do with the big issues and debates, the ethics of corporate sponsorship, raising money or finding the cure, and all to do with personal connection and acknowledgment, where "small" acts are the ones that matter. These are of such importance, way more than all the rhetoric and reasoning and public fights, because ultimately it is a personal battle.

"One of the most profound responses to breast cancer today is the gathering of women together, but by very definition, the experience of breast cancer is a solitary one," Iona Campagnolo, Lieutenant-Governor of British Columbia, said in her opening remarks at the Third World Breast Cancer Conference in Victoria in 2002.[30] She is right on both counts. "When women connect with other women and become part of a community of people who are going through [breast cancer] and feeling the same fear and confusion and self-doubt and anger, . . . there is an incredibly powerful light that goes on and when that gets channelled into action, watch out because it can be formidable."[31]

It might seem, however, that beneath the rhetoric and the rallying cries, the networking and jockeying, you are still alone with a disease for which there is no cure yet. In the middle of the night, the chorus of all the voices speaking out may be silenced by your own—a solitary plea that you will survive long enough until one is found.

It is comforting, though, that when you surface from your personal struggle, you find a whole army of women who have "been there," along with their families and friends, working for change. They are working for you. "Advocacy creates a community where the voices of all affected women can be heard."[32] Even if you yourself are not speaking out loud, but just whimpering softly in the night.

8 | THE OTHER SHOE: METASTATIC DISEASE

It has become, in my view, a bit too trendy to regard the acceptance of death as something tantamount to intrinsic dignity. Of course I agree with the preacher of Ecclesiastes that there is a time to love and a time to die—and when my skein runs out I hope to face the end calmly and in my own way. For most situations, however, I prefer the more martial view that death is the ultimate enemy—and I find nothing reproachable in those who rage mightily against the dying of the light.

—Stephen Jay Gould, "The Median Isn't the Message"[1]

THIS TIME the phone call was from Scott. "It's bad news," he said. "It's the worst it can be."

Nicole's cancer was back, everywhere. They had just seen her oncologist: a CT scan and a lung biopsy indicated clusters of nodules in her lungs, cancer in her hip and on the chest wall. She had no breasts for it to come back in, so it erupted on the sternum. It was April 2000, three years after her initial diagnosis.

There had been clues earlier. She developed a persistent hacking cough in February, and it was Scott who finally said, "You've had this cough for a month now, maybe you should get a chest film, maybe you've got pneumonia or something."

"She had no pain, she was just coughing a lot. We weren't even thinking of metastatic disease. During that period from Christmas of '97 she was in good shape," Scott says. "She didn't dwell on the cancer . . . I think she thought, that was then, this is now."[2]

It was on her youngest daughter Saraya's fifth birthday when Nicole received the initial results of the X-rays: "multiple densities: suggest CT scan." She took the X-rays to her oncologist, who didn't see any densities and thought that the radiologist had "over-read" the film. So she went back to radiology and asked a resident to look at the film. She recounted the conversation:

"'I was just discussing this case with Dr. X,' I told the resident, 'and . . .'"

"'That density is not the only thing going on in this X-ray,' the resident interrupts. 'This patient definitely needs a CT.'"

"'I was just on my way to organizing that for her,' I say in a small voice."

Not admitting that she was the patient who had the busy X-ray.

She had the CT scan that evening, which confirmed that nothing had been over-read: at least 20 nodules, the radiologist said; it's almost certain to be cancer. She called her oncologist from the clinic, but he still wasn't convinced. He advised a lung biopsy because "we really have to make the fat lady sing here, Nicole."

A week later she had a laparoscopic thoracotomy (biopsy of the lung, a painful invasive procedure that requires a general anaesthetic). When she woke up in the recovery room, the first thing Nicole heard was one nurse saying to another that the local anaesthetic that was supposed to be dripping into her, into the intrapleural space, had not yet arrived from the pharmacy.

"I was in agony . . . [but] more agonizing was not knowing the results of the biopsy. I was transferred to my room and Scott gave me the news. I was devastated."

The next morning she had an MRI, which confirmed the metasta-sis to the hip. The chest tube was removed and she was sent home on Good Friday. She spent Easter weekend in a psychological daze, "a major snake pit," as she put it.

When Nicole had finished her treatment the first time around and regained her health, her hair, her strength, she went back to work, she joined the Ottawa breast cancer dragon-boat team and she threw herself into investigating and speaking out about the impact of chem-ical pesticides on human health, particularly the health of children. "She really had to know what the hell had caused her cancer," Scott says. "She looked at the classical risk factors for breast cancer and she was casting around asking, How come I got it? I tried to explain to her that there is such a thing as pure bad luck. But she had to have a reason, and I initially didn't understand that, but I grew to understand that she had to have something to hang her hat on, to be able to say, 'This is the reason I got breast cancer.'"

During that time, she lived life to the fullest, drawing on her personal experience with the disease as well as her credentials as a highly respected physician in her community to make people listen: she did not have the breast cancer gene (she had been tested earlier on—it doesn't matter for me, she said, but she wanted to know for her daughters), she had taken the recommended treatments, all of them, without complaint, she had had a second mastectomy; she shouldn't have gotten the bloody disease in the first place, and now this.

❧

At the Third World Conference on Breast Cancer, about 800 delegates "converged" on Victoria, B.C. That's how the crawl across the bottom of the TV screen of CBC Newsworld put it, conveying the impression of locusts arriving to devour a crop called breast cancer.

For most delegates, this was not an academic exercise; they came to seek and give information on a topic that seared their hearts. The vast majority were women—women with breast cancer, women who had had breast cancer and women who were afraid they would get breast cancer. Perhaps the greatest number were those who, having endured a first go-round with the disease, and the accompanying battery of treatments, were now in that in-between world, fearful of hearing the other shoe drop.

Vladana Sistek was there. She had come from Brockville, Ontario, signing on as a volunteer. Her breast cancer diagnosis had been in March 2001, a little more than a year earlier. "I went to the conference to get more information. It was odd for me because all previous conferences I'd gone to as a professional to get information to help me deal with patients. But at this one—I was the patient."[3]

Vladana is a psychiatric social worker. She was 39 years old, a single parent with two boys, when she found the lump in her breast while showering. "It was a bolt out of the blue. I'm an avid squash player, sometimes showering twice a day, and never felt it, then suddenly it was there." A three-centimetre lump.

"Fourteen years of social work had in some ways prepared me for dealing with this. I knew all the stages of grief; I knew I was supposed to be angry, depressed and then was to reach acceptance, so I don't think I had as much of the emotional shock or initial devastation of having that first diagnosis. I knew what to expect."

Vladana had a mastectomy and node excision, which indicated that five nodes were cancerous. "I was offered a [clinical] trial. After I agreed to go in, I was randomly assigned to one of the arms of the trial. I had chemotherapy and radiation and then I thought I would be fine. . . . The chemotherapy I was on in the clinical trial was very aggressive; my blood count went down to almost nothing, I had to go on Neupogen [a drug that stimulates the white blood cells] and also antibiotics. Given the aggressivity of that treatment, it did not occur to [me] that there might be metastasis. At the conference I didn't go to any of the sessions on metastasis because I thought 'I'm not there, I don't need to know that . . .' Never dawned on me whatsoever that the cancer might metastasize."

At the conference, Vladana was plagued with a pain in her arm and shoulder; she went into a walk-in clinic in Victoria and was told it was bursitis. When she got home, she went to her own doctor and was told the same thing. "When I asked the doctor if it could be the cancer back, he said no. He scheduled me for physiotherapy but did ask for X-rays."

The X-rays showed another three-centimetre tumour, this time on her humerus. A bone scan showed that the cancer was also in the pelvic and lumbar region. Ultrasound found lesions on her liver. Her oncologist said, "The dirty little bastards got away from the chemo."

Metastatic disease—the stuff of nightmares. The enemy that you thought, you hoped, you prayed had been vanquished, is back. Every woman who has had breast cancer fears recurrence because it flips you across the border from "curable" to "chronic," euphemisms that describe a disease that is curable as long as it doesn't come back and chronic as long as your body can tolerate a sequential battery of treatments and the cancer cells can't.

The word "cancer" strikes terror, cloaked as it is in centuries of lore. When yoked with the word "metastatic," the terror is compounded. The fearful trappings and persona of all stages of breast cancer have been pushed onto metastatic, because cure really isn't in the picture. The current lingo describes women with metastatic disease as "living with cancer," as if it's a tame and tidy pet curled up on the hearth, needing an occasional meal and a pat on the head, rather than a wild and badly trained carnivore chewing away in your body, a junkyard dog wearing you down with its ravenous and erratic presence. "We can't predict the course of any individual's illness. This is true of initial disease, and metastatic disease is even more unpredictable."[4]

It used to be that a breast cancer diagnosis carried a stigma that imprisoned women in fear and shame and silence. In the last couple of decades, that has changed, at least in North America and Europe. A confluence of elements has brought breast cancer very much into the public eye. The stigma has gone. Or has it? Many women feel that it has simply been shifted down the line: a primary diagnosis is okay, people around you can deal with it; a diagnosis of metastatic disease is not, because it comes with the spectre of imminent death. Metastatic disease is still the bogeyman, kept in the closet by the cheery messages dominating public awareness and fundraising campaigns. The reality is cloaked in a pink mantle of denial spun from carefully worded slogans such as "Breast cancer can be beaten." They hedge their bets in a semantic thicket of future and conditional tense, but the intended message, couched in relentless optimism, is that no one dies of this disease. But the harsh message is that they do. This obfuscation masks a more important message: that the diagnosis of metastatic disease does not mean "The End." It is understandable that the public might not know this, given that the media don't talk about metastatic disease much, but it is discouraging when doctors don't seem to know it either.

When Valerie Whyte was diagnosed with advanced cancer—stage 4—following a hip fracture, she was referred to an oncologist, who would tell her the next steps. He pretty much told her there were none, and not just because her hip had disintegrated.

"I now understand that he was writing me off because I was metastatic, too late for anything but palliative care," Valerie says. "Luckily for me, when my surgeon heard that, he hit the ceiling—he more or less made me get a second opinion, and the second oncologist said, no, you have a good chance. His attitude was that, 'We're going to fight this and prolong your life and make sure you have a decent quality of life.'"[5]

Valerie encountered others in the medical profession who thought that people with metastatic disease had lost the battle: "When you are diagnosed with primary cancer, the doctors try to cure you, and if it doesn't work, then too bad, so sad. . . . We might as well go away and die somewhere. So thank goodness for that surgeon; thank goodness for Sheila [Valerie's sister], who, as soon as she heard 'second opinion,' took control of me and said, 'Right, let's go.'"

Nicole once told a friend who also had advanced disease, "When I was in medical school, I was taught, for people like us, just to keep them comfortable and send them off to palliative care. Ingrid, don't let yourself buy into *that* theory. We have to swim against the stream."[6] Women with metastatic breast cancer are swimming against the stream like never before, and living longer and better for it. Even the statistics are encouraging: "Fully 20 percent of newly diagnosed metastatic breast cancer patients live five years or more."[7] There seems to be a combination of reasons: improvement in treatment; a new understanding of the impact of physical exercise on extension and quality of life; and recognition of the importance of the intangibles—psychosocial support from health care professionals, patients, peers and family.

❧

Metastasis, from the Greek, means "removal." In cancer, it is the spreading of cancer cells from the primary site through the lymphatic or blood systems to other sites in the body. Musa Meyer, author and breast cancer survivor, writes, "The process of metastasis isn't random . . . it is a cascade of linked sequential steps that must be traversed by the tumor cells . . . To be successful, a metastatic tumor cell must leave the primary tumor and invade local host tissue. It must then enter the circulation, survive in the circulation, arrest at the distant vascular bed, extravasate (or spread) into the organ interstitium (space between the organs) and/or parenchyma (the organ itself). . . ."[8] In other words, it goes forth and multiplies.

Micrometastases—seeds from the primary tumour—are too tiny to be picked up on a bone scan or any blood test, including those done after a primary diagnosis to establish baseline data. Your doctor will probably tell you this at the time. Mine did, but the information didn't stick. So fogged by the initial diagnosis, I could barely grasp the concept of metastasis, let alone pronounce it; micrometastases floated right by me. Which is what they do in the body, undetected, undetectable, like tiny seed pods waiting for spring. Sometimes they lie dormant for years or forever; sometimes they blossom and grow with alarming speed. They are, everyone agrees, unpredictable. Why does one person's cancer remain quiescent, another person's cancer grow like a weed?

Darwin has given us part of the answer, his insight that, "among members of a species, what is important is not the similarities but the differences."[9] Here is the tripwire for those looking for blanket therapies, national treatment guidelines and standard one-size-fits-all approaches to curing cancer. But it also provides the threshold of hope for the human spirit: unpredictability and differences mean each woman can hope to be the one with quiescent cancer cells and not weeds.

Metastasis can come in a variety of ways. All recurrences are usually lumped in under metastatic disease, but there are degrees of recurrence. Some can be put in a kind of subcategory, more serious than a primary diagnosis and less problematic than a metastatic diagnosis. Sounds picky, but it's one of those important details that can be a comfort when you are trying to figure out whether it was a slipper or a full metal boot that has dropped.

Local recurrence is when cancer cells grow again at the primary site, forming another tumour. Regional recurrence, considered more serious, is tumour growth on the muscles of the chest wall, the mammary lymph nodes under the breastbone and between the ribs, the nodes in the neck and above the collarbone.

Then there is distant recurrence, which is serious metastasis, when cancer cells colonize in bone (accounting for 75 percent of recurrence) and vital—"vital" as in necessary to live—organs of the body, the lungs and liver usually. Or as my oncologist put it, "Breast cancer likes bone, brain, lungs and liver." Like that junkyard dog settling down to dinner.

The early symptoms of recurrence are tough to distinguish from so many other, much more benign, changes in your body. When you've had cancer once, though, it is difficult to believe with any certainty that a fleeting pain, a swollen joint, even a bad cold is anything but the cancer come back. "Once you are diagnosed with cancer, your life is never the same. We can no longer have a headache from stress—**It's** going to the brain. We can no longer have a backache from sleeping on the wrong side—**It's** in the bones."[10]

Several years after I finished treatment, I developed a lump on my foot behind the bunion bone. It was painful and did not go away. Eventually my GP referred me to an orthopaedic surgeon, a small, tough, no-nonsense kind of guy who obviously thought I was wasting his time. When I told him that I'd had breast cancer and was still and always watchful for lumps, anywhere, he was dismissive. "You don't get cancer of the foot," he snapped.

Well, what did I know? There are bones in the feet, aren't there? (And as it turns out, according to another doctor, you *can* get bone metastasis to the foot—rarely, but it happens.) My foot lump wasn't cancer, it was a ganglion—a cyst on the nerve. It's still there, and it still hurts. But it's astonishing how fast your mind recalibrates your body's response to pain when you know it isn't cancer again. Perspective is everything.

It helps though if you can at least restrict your worry to the more likely sites and symptoms for recurrence. "If you know that the symptoms of breast cancer metastasis are usually bone pain, shortness of breath, lack of appetite and weight loss, and neurological symptoms like pain or weakness or headaches, there are at least limits to your fear."[11] So what else is there? Well, there's abdominal pain, a persistent cough, a skin rash . . . Fear can rattle around pretty much at will within such broad parameters.

The "R" word—recurrence—strikes terror in your heart. Once you've had breast cancer, it lurks like Banquo's ghost, ready to sit right down at the dinner table again. But does it help to keep constant vigilance, poised to act instantly if you catch it sidling into a chair? Musa Meyer, who wrote *Advanced Breast Cancer: A Guide to Living with Metastatic Disease,* says there is a myth about early detection of metastasis. We are cautioned to be ever watchful, have X-rays, scans, blood tests, the whole battery of tools that make up the DEW Line barrier of recurrence. Even if advanced disease is found early, does it make a difference? She says not. Detecting metastasis before symptoms appear does not improve survival or quality of life: "There is no early detection for metastatic breast cancer because it's not early when you find it."[12]

"This is not a message of hopelessness," she says. That would be the worst message to take away with you. Recurrence is not an immediate death sentence. "Widely disseminated metastatic breast cancer is among the most treatable of advanced cancers." What she is saying is that screening X-rays and scans to detect early metastasis are both unreliable and unnecessary. Eighty-five percent of breast cancer metastasis is discovered by physical exam and patient history alone: the far more efficient detection method is the old-fashioned one: talk to your doctor about any possible symptoms.

Meyer says that she at first rejected this idea as low-tech and quaint but eventually was convinced by her research: one large study showed that of 11,000 follow-up chest X-rays of women who had had breast cancer, exactly one lung metastasis was found in patients who hadn't had any other symptoms. Another study of the efficacy of follow-up testing, including bone scans, tumour markers and liver function tests, found that after 10 years, there was no difference in survival time between the group that had these tests and the group that didn't. A meta-analysis of four trials on follow-up strategies came up with the same results. Conclusion: a physical examination was better than all the fancy tests. The Canadian Medical Association endorses this approach, recommending that routine laboratory and radiographic investigations should not be carried out for the purposes of detecting distant metastasis.[13]

You could look on this recommendation as an indictment of medical scientific technology, or you could embrace what Meyer calls the "paradox of powerlessness." After she learned of these studies, she said, "It was such a relief, I was free to go on with my life relieved of the burden of vigilance. I learned from women living with recurrence [that] there is no real preparation for that kind of bad news. . . . There can be power in giving up the need to control what cannot be controlled."

This does not mean you should ignore symptoms. Trust your body to tell you if something is wrong; listen to it and make sure your doctor is listening to you. Some women report a lot of deafness in the medical profession when it comes to matters of recurrence. "Every time you get an ache or a pain that lasts a little bit longer than normal," one woman reported, "the first place that you go to in your head, after you have had a diagnosis, is whether the cancer's back. I find that doctors don't want to hear about this."[14] So yell a lot.

Treatments for metastatic disease are similar to those for primary, only more so and with exceptions. If you already have had radiation treatment to a breast, you cannot have it again to that same part of your body. And chemotherapy is usually, though not always, stronger. It is impossible to do more than generalize here, because there are so many approaches—depending on the tumour type, site and aggressiveness—and by the time you read this, there could be a whole lot more. Of the smorgasbord of options, which one you are offered depends in large part on your doctor. This is often difficult to accept, because we want to believe that there is one best way to beat the disease. There isn't. We look for certainty; we'd be content with consensus. What we perceive is confusion. A positive spin on this is yes, there *is* confusion, but only because the treatment choices are so much greater than they were a few years ago. Exactly because there are so many approaches being investigated, physicians must make choices, and they must base their choices on their own knowledge of the research, their observations of responses in their patients, their preference for clinical trials or standard approaches and, finally, their personal biases formed who knows where or why.

Of course, there are guidelines, and there are indications from your specific situation that influence your doctor's recommendation. If, however, you consult other doctors, especially if they practise in different cancer centres, you could easily get different recommendations. "One doctor may want to put you on hormone therapy, another may want to add combination chemotherapy to the hormonal treatment, still another may suggest you might be a candidate for dose-dense chemotherapy on its own. This doesn't mean that these doctors don't know what they are talking about, only that, given the available information, they have drawn different conclusions about how to proceed."[15] It is, nevertheless, unnerving, and it reinforces the conclusion of many women that it's all a crapshoot, just the luck of the draw not only who gets breast cancer but who gets the "right" therapy and who survives breast cancer whatever the treatment. In the meantime, what you do is work hard to load the dice in your favour.

"Confusing and disturbing as conflicting recommendations may be, they also suggest that control over your treatment is in your hands, and that the choice, ultimately, is yours to make," writes Meyer.[16] For some women, this is a particularly threatening concept, trailing with it the fear and guilt of making the wrong choice. For other women, the sense of personal control is as empowering as the therapy itself might be.

Shail Verma, oncologist at the Ottawa Regional Cancer Centre, agrees. A patient of his had been told that her cancer may have spread: "Her immediate reaction was one of incredible wrath, not directed at anyone, just that this had happened. . . . I had a letter from her saying, 'I'm going for another CAT scan and [if the metastasis is confirmed], I'm going away; I'm going to cash in my RRSPs and live out my life and then when I run out of money I'll come back and see you.' I thought, gosh, you know, this is a woman who can get the most coveted drug in breast cancer therapy—Herceptin—because her tumour would respond to that drug, and she won't take it. I thought to myself, I could try and talk some sense into her, [but] on the other hand, there is so much of life that needs to be lived. What would I do? Part of me would want to run away and live my life, too. Is that a wrong thing or a right thing? I don't know. I think the individual needs to have the freedom of that choice, but they must have the freedom to return without recrimination on either side—oh look, you let me go off and look where I'm at, or, no, I don't want to see you, bye. That freedom of choice and access availability need to be underlined."[17]

So, you might choose to do nothing, or you might choose to abandon the conventional route and look for alternative approaches, or you might follow one of the paths carved out by clinical trials. No one, absolutely no one, can say which is the right way for you. Except you.

A diagnosis of primary breast cancer—or "early breast cancer," as it's often called, a term suggesting that "late cancer" can't be far behind—is a frightful shock, partly because you don't feel sick. How could you have cancer and still feel fine? Then you don't feel so fine, but it's the treatment that turns you into a sick person, that provides the tangible proof that, at least for a time, you are living in the kingdom of the ill. With advanced cancer, the disease itself makes its presence known, has moved out of the breast, eventually to interfere with the functions of whatever organ or bone structure it has colonized. For many patients at this stage, treatment is no longer the enemy but an ally in fighting the disease. "However arduous, the treatment becomes associated with hope, and from that hope flows the strength to endure the treatments."[18]

Since by definition metastatic cancer is systemic, surgery and radiation, which are localized treatments, are less effective than they are for primary cancer. Both, however, are used extensively for palliative and supportive care with metastatic disease. Radiation is used to relieve pain, to reduce tumour pressure on vital organs or nerves, to prevent tumour growth and broken bones. Surgery is used for biopsies, mastectomies, oophorectomies, to implant portocatheters and to debulk large tumours. A surgical procedure is used to insert a tube into the pleural cavity (the space enclosed by the pleura tissue covering the lungs and lining of the chest cavity) and the pericardial cavity (the sac around the heart) to drain off malignant fluid. Nicole had this procedure done dozens and dozens of times, sometimes up to three times a week, to reduce the fierce pressure on her lungs and her heart caused by constant fluid build-up.

Evidence-based medicine has put hormonal therapies and chemotherapies, and most recently biological or targetted therapies (see introduction) at the forefront in treatment of metastatic disease, but within those categories, there are myriad choices. Hormonal therapies are the standard for hormone-positive tumours; chemotherapy, for hormone-negative tumours. But there's a catch. Tumours that tested hormone-positive at first diagnosis aren't necessarily hormone-positive the second time around, and vice versa. Indeed, in one study, "36 percent of estrogen [hormone]-positive tumors following first diagnosis were no longer positive at the time of recurrence."[19]

Chemotherapies range from high-dose to low-dose to dose-dense, from oral to infusion, from highly toxic to palliative. High-dose chemo, a term usually used to describe a bone marrow transplant followed by high doses of chemo, seems to have proven ineffective, although this approach is still in clinical trials, particularly in the United States. A few years ago, it was touted as the answer, but "it seems proven to be a misdirection," says oncologist Shail Verma. "These are incredibly awful toxic drugs, and there's a certain threshold beyond which the body will not accept them." Researchers are starting to arrive at this conclusion; women on high-dose treatments knew this a long time ago.

"In advanced cancer," Musa Meyer writes, "'dose intensity' strategies like high-dose chemotherapy have shown clear limitations, thus 'throwing doubt on the assertion that optimal cytotoxic therapy can kill all tumor cells.'"[20] "Cytotoxic" is the medical equivalent to the military term "collateral damage": cytotoxic drugs batter healthy cells as well as cancer cells.

But dose-dense chemotherapy, which is governed by a similar "big stick" philosophy, is receiving a lot of excited support, based on the results of one large study of 2,000 patients. "Dose-dense" simply means taking standard drugs in a shorter time frame. In the study, all patients were given the standard combination of Adriamycin, Taxol and Cytoxan but according to different regimens. The results indicated that those who were given the drugs every two weeks instead of every three fared better. Definition of "fared better": disease-free survival after four years was 82 percent in the group on the dose-dense regimen, 75 percent in the group on the conventional regimen. "In addition to improved disease-free survival, the study indicated that dose-dense chemotherapy may also lead to higher overall survival rates. After three years, 92 percent of patients on the dose-dense therapy were alive, compared to 90 percent of those on the conventionally administered regimens."[21]

"This study suggests that many women with breast cancer may benefit from chemotherapy administered on a condensed schedule," says Dr. Marc L. Citron, the lead investigator of the study. "With the availability of new drugs to control one of the most serious side effects of chemotherapy administration, we can further increase the chances of survival for women with breast cancer." By further increasing the intensity of the chemotherapy, "the dose dense regimen was made tolerable for patients because of the drug filgrastim [Neupogen], which helps prevent neutropenia [low white blood cell count], a serious complication of chemotherapy."[22]

Two points here. First, Neupogen is very expensive, more than the cost of the three chemotherapy drugs combined. For women without a private drug plan, the prohibitive cost of Neupogen puts it out of reach of most. Even if you are participating in a clinical trial, in most jurisdictions the cost of such non-chemo drugs is not covered. If you have a drug plan, you probably would receive partial coverage. (When Vladana was on an aggressive chemotherapy regimen within a trial, her medical plan covered 80 percent of the cost of the Neupogen.)

Second, the body is still taking a tough battering on this regimen, even though the symptoms of it might be masked by such drugs as Neupogen. However, the doctors in charge of the study claim that the side effects are not as bad as with standard treatment. Other oncologists agree with this assessment. Dr. Verma says, "Women have a lot of fatigue and blood effects, but paradoxically, when you compare them with effects of [standard regimens], they have fewer complications." However, some women on the receiving end don't completely agree.

One patient, who is also a doctor, chose to take part in a clinical study of dose-dense chemo: "Before consenting, I read the actual research protocol, in addition to the one usually given to patients. I thought I knew what the words nausea, fatigue, fever, chills, low blood counts, shortness of breath, bone pain and trouble swallowing meant. When I experienced them myself, I saw how very little I had really comprehended. . . . As the protocol proceeded, I got sicker and sicker."[23] She ended up in hospital nine times because of neutropenia and fever.

Dr. Larry Norton of the Memorial Sloan-Kettering Cancer Center says, "If confirmed with additional research, this approach may change the standard of care in breast cancer treatment."[24] At least one previous study did not show the same positive results, and it is discouraging that the "standard" in treatment might become more, rather than less, damaging to the rest of the body.

Other research points in a quite different direction: that all cells in a tumour are not equally malignant and that only a tiny minority actually induce new cancers; the rest are relatively harmless. In a lab experiment in which tumours were induced in mice, it appeared that while all the cells in the original tumours replicated themselves, as few as 100 to 200 out of tens of thousands actually caused more tumour growth in the animals. "In the light of these findings, strategies that aim at simply shrinking tumors with radiation or chemotherapy are doomed to failure."[25] Ouch.

According to Max S. Wicha, an oncologist and director of the University of Michigan Comprehensive Cancer Center, this is why current treatments for metastatic breast cancer often fail. "The goal of all our existing therapies has been to kill as many cells within the tumor as possible, [but these findings] suggest that the current model may not be getting us anywhere, because we have been targeting the wrong cells with the wrong treatments. . . . [Now] we can define what we believe are the important cells, the cells which determine whether the cancer will come back or be cured. . . . Before this, we didn't even know there were such cells."[26]

Another example of "Watch this space." In the meantime, an encouraging development in improving the quality of life of metastatic patients, whichever treatment they choose, is the use of bone strengtheners. Dr. Verma says that this is one of the most heartening directions in treatment of metastatic disease: "The pamidronates and other drugs that protect the bones [ensure that] women don't go through all those awful complications . . . fractured hips or fractured spines."

With the discovery of the tumour in her shoulder, Vladana had localized radiation treatments and started hormone treatment, but they weren't working. She was rapidly getting much worse. "My movement was restricted, I could not get up easily; it was like I had lost all my muscles. Even to turn over in bed I needed help—the cancer is all down my back and in my leg—it just progressed, continued to get worse." A new bone scan and ultrasound showed spread throughout her body, and now her oncologist was pushing hard for chemotherapy.

"I had been resisting [chemo]," Vladana says, "because . . . it didn't work the first time, although I was told, well, maybe it did work, because if I hadn't taken it, I might be in much worse shape now. I suppose it is quite possible that it slowed down the progression." Her doctor also put her on a bone strengthener (clodronate), which he described as super glue for the bones. "I decided that was for me . . .

super glue would be good"; her bones seemed to be weakening by the minute. Vladana did some research on another drug, pamidronate, an infusion that looked as if it might be more effective. She asked her doctor if she could try it, but even though the drug had been approved for bone metastasis, he couldn't give it to her.

"A lot of these drugs you can get if you're symptomatic, but not before," she says. "But I don't want the symptoms; why can't I have these drugs as preventative? The doctor said he couldn't [prescribe them], his hands were tied; he tried to get the drug for me, but was told no. He said, 'You're talking to the converted—I spend 70 percent of my time trying to persuade the powers that be to allow me to prescribe certain drugs.'"

Valerie Whyte was given pamidronate, but *after* her hip shattered, which it did for no apparent reason. She had started to have X-rays and tests to see what was wrong because the pain in her back and hip was growing more and more severe. "I've never experienced that kind of pain before, but of course it was a stress fracture, [my hip] was full of hairline fractures, and then it fell apart. I was getting into my car in the car port and I just fell to the ground." She fell because her hip broke, not the other way around.

Valerie was treated in the orthopaedic ward, and it wasn't until the doctors put pins in to hold her joint in place that they discovered what had caused it to shatter. It was riddled and eaten through by cancer, cancer that had started in the breast.

"Most of the people [in my support group] were first diagnosed with primary cancer and then five, six, seven, eight, nine years later were diagnosed with metastatic, and it was a terrible blow, even worse the second time; this was a blow that I didn't have to deal with because it all happened at once," she explains with irony.

Valerie had noticed a very small lump in her breast six months before but didn't do anything about it. These were the last few months of her father's life; he was dying of Alzheimer's disease, and she was going flat out, juggling the pieces of her life in not enough time to keep even some of them in the air. "I blame myself a little bit. I know there's absolutely no point in doing so but I recognize my responsibility. . . . I kept postponing my doctor's appointments. . . . If I had taken care of it earlier, I might not have had a broken hip, although the oncologist said I probably would already have had bone metastasis. . . . But you know, I chalk that up to life. Breast cancer can operate like that [she slaps her hands together]; it can be in the body for 10 years and then, wham, it's gone into the lymph nodes and the bones so fast."

Valerie had chemotherapy—very aggressive chemotherapy—before surgery to shrink the tumour. "My oncologist . . . was very clear about what he was going to give me, how many chemo treatments, how much my body could stand, and I would have to have ECGs [to monitor the possible damage to her heart]. He was very clear about the dangers of it. The chemo took about four hours to administer, on Friday, then on the Monday, a two-hour top up. Every three weeks." After every treatment, her oncologist would get out his tape measure and measure the tumour and say, "It's getting smaller and smaller, so you must be doing something right."

"The first eight months of my illness," Valerie says, "I was dealing with the chemo and a broken hip, which of course never healed because of the chemo. I couldn't put any weight on my leg and had to travel back and forth to [the hospital for chemotherapy] by ambulance." After six months, she asked her orthopaedic surgeon when he was going to tell her she could put weight on her hip. "Why don't you try it now," he said. "The worst thing that can happen, it could fall apart, and if it does, we'll give you a new one."

About a year and a half after diagnosis and eight months after the end of chemo, Valerie had a hip replacement, and this time it worked. "It has been wonderful." Then she adds with understatement, "The pins in my hip did *not* work." She could actually feel them pulling apart during the four months she had to wait for the operation.

"I have diffuse bone mets [metastasis], which means it's pretty much everywhere, like salt," Valerie says. "I have generalized bone pain when I get cold or tired, also I'm on a continuing medication—pamidronate," the bone strengthener that Vladana tried unsuccessfully to get. Valerie's oncologist prescribed it at the beginning of her treatment, at the same time as chemo. He told her that he didn't know if it would help, that all he knew, from observation, was that patients who took it fared better than patients who didn't.

"I believe it helps," Valerie says. "They've found lots more evidence that not only is it effective in building up bones but that it is effective in beating back cancer. It prevents cancer cells from moving into weakened areas or something. . . . I have been able to rebuild the strength in my bones. It also acts as a pain control."

Vladana had been on the right track. Some bone strengtheners, including the one her doctor *could* prescribe for her, are in clinical trials for treatment following primary or early breast cancer. The results are promising. Some research is suggesting that drugs such as clodronate, originally used to treat osteoporosis, might even help to prevent bone metastasis.[27]

The bone strengtheners are only one of the positive developments in metastatic breast cancer treatment. "I've been working for two decades in breast cancer, and I can tell you," Shail Verma says, "when I started, if a woman had metastatic disease anywhere other than bone, she was dead in a year. Today, our clinics are crammed with women with metastatic disease who are surviving and surviving and surviving, and doing reasonably well. I attribute this to an intelligent use of sequential therapy. You have one treatment that stops working because it gets resistant, then you move to another one and then to another one, and another. We have a lot more tools."

Valerie is working her way through the sequence, surviving and surviving and surviving. Because her tumour was estrogen-positive, she was put on tamoxifen, "which did quite a lot of good for almost two years before it stopped working," she says. "But the bone lesions started to grow again and now I am on Femara. I've been on it for

15 months, but now there are new spots and some of those are getting bigger. . . . My present oncologist thinks that if Femara stops working, there are other things that we can try. Her attitude is that every couple of years there are new things to try. It's an attitude I can live with. It's bought me almost two years. . . ."

Valerie also has another theory about her ability to survive this far: "Partly it's me, my personality—I felt very optimistic about my treatment. . . . From the very beginning I thought if I don't get any worse, I can stand this and I can get better, not better as in fully recuperate, but just better than I was then—and that's been the case. My physical condition and my quality of life have improved in the last year and a half. And that's been very encouraging. . . . I see the last three and a half years as a kind of a gift. My condition is not going away, but I feel much better, physically I feel much better as time goes on. But the cancer is progressing; every time I have a bone scan there are more and more spots, but I'm not suffering for it and everything seems to have really slowed down. As we say in my group, bone mets doesn't kill you. It [does] when it goes into the liver, brain and lungs. So far so good."

Valerie's group is made up of people with metastatic cancer; they are the embodiment of survivorship. They talk about cancer as controllable, not terminal. Even though their bodies may be shot through with disease, their spirits soar, or struggle, depending on the day, but they are there for each other always. "We all get such great pleasure out of each other's victories," Valerie says, a powerful expression of the connection within what she calls her "new circle of friends," a circle of hope.

9 BEYOND STATISTICS: THE LONG RIGHT TAIL OF HOPE

Hope is the space between symptoms and diagnosis, between diagnosis and prognosis. It is the wrestling match between science and compassion; between body and spirit, between pain and relief. . . . Hoping is being treated, not as another case of a particular disease, but as a person. . . . Hoping is denying the statistics. Reaching beyond the traditional. Keeping open the possibility of being the exception. Hoping is listening to the unconscious. Having dreams in the world of sleep and dreams in the world of consciousness.

—Ronna Jayne, "Hope and Illness"[1]

WHEN HER ONCOLOGIST CONFIRMED that her cancer was back, Nicole was shattered. Not only by the news but by how he delivered it. "He talked to her not as to a patient but as he would to another physician," Scott says. "I remember exactly, he told her that the median survival time for somebody with her presentation now, the median time for disease progression under this regimen of Taxotere, is 10 months. I'm convinced that he would never have said that to another patient, a non-physician patient."[2]

Nicole said, flatly, "He took away my hope." The medium was the message. The Doctor was Death. What she could not see, through the veil of fear, was that the *median* was not the message. Nicole knew what the odds were because she was a physician and had breast cancer patients and had seen what could happen to them; she didn't delude herself as to what she faced.

She wrote down what she remembered of the conversation. This was the oncologist who had said to her a few days before, hoping against hope that what was showing up in her lung X-ray was not cancer, that the fat lady was not singing yet. "Well, the fat lady is singing now," she told him.

"Yes, I know, and I want you to know Nicole that I am very sorry about it. I also know of no therapy conventional or alternative in North America or Europe that will cure metastatic breast cancer." Nicole said she didn't hear much after that. "Of course I know *that* at an intellectual level too, but as to why it had to be explicitly laid out to me then in that way is still beyond me. [I am writing this] several months later and I am firmly convinced that these few words have been the most damaging thing that has happened to my health, including the cancer."

Perhaps her oncologist thought that because she was a doctor she would not interpret the information he gave her as a non-doctor would; that a median mortality of 10 months, she'd understand, did not mean that she would die in 10 months; that, with her training in statistics, she would know that the median is a measure of central tendency, and that the reality lies in the variation from it. If this had been an intellectual medical discussion, an abstract debate around the family dinner table, Nicole would have argued that this was not a prognostic certainty for individual patients but a statistical basket of data. Now though, it was way too close to home.

The cancer that had physically taken over her lungs and bones, figuratively took over her brain, her well-honed powers of reasoning and perspective. Under the circumstances, it was impossible for her to extrapolate the information she needed most, to recognize that for statistics to set the mortality median at 10 months, half the people in the equation had to be on the right side of the median line, people who live longer than 10 months. She could be one of those.

In his essay "The Median Isn't the Message," Stephen Jay Gould writes about his own eight-month mortality median prognosis after being diagnosed with abdominal mesothelioma, a cancer associated with asbestos exposure. Instead of being felled by the gloomy statistics, he offers his personal view that statistics, when "properly interpreted," can be "profoundly nurturant and life-giving."[3]

"Statistics recognize different measures of an 'average,' or central tendency," Gould writes. "The *mean* is our usual concept of an overall average—add up the items and divide them by the number of sharers. . . . The *median,* a different measure of central tendency, is the half-way point." This means that half the people with this disease live past the halfway point. So, what are the chances of my being in that half? he asked himself. They were pretty good—he was young, he would receive the best medical treatment available; "I had the world to live for." Another source of comfort was his recognition that the distribution of the variation about the median was right skewed. In his case, the left side has to be scrunched up between zero and eight months, but the right side can extend out for years, the long right tail beyond the median, the long right tail of hope.

Another mesothelioma patient I met had an oncologist who seemed to have succumbed to an obsession with the mean so utterly that he forgot that "the 'average person' is a mathematical construct, corresponding to no actual human being."[4] He told his patient, "Fifty percent of people with your cancer die in the first year after diagnosis. Fifty percent die in the second year," thus neatly lopping off the right tail to match the left. But, and this is so important, in individual cases, the part of the graph line to the right of the median does not necessarily mirror the left side; as Gould points out, it is often right skewed. The median prognosis is based on a collection of data averaged from a population of patients with the cancer in question. Some individuals might not make it to the median, others, like Gould, survive way past it. This patient was already inching out beyond the median. He was in a wheelchair, his skin liverish and mottled, but not his spirit: "It's a good day today," he said cheerfully, "because, hey, I'm still above ground."

Statistics can be toppled. Statistics are mindless, heartless, soulless number-crunching entities, as stupid in their way as genes. They can't compute the human spirit, the anomalies, the variables, the unknowns. They can't dictate who is on the right side of the median, who gets to sit at the end of the long tail. And they certainly can't measure or account for the power of hope.

⁓

Valerie Whyte's first oncologist was also caught in the web of statistical prognoses; he gave her the impression that there was no hope—she did have stage 4 breast cancer after all; luckily, her second oncologist saw past both the statistics and the disease to the person beyond. "He gave me a lot of encouragement and compassion, and whatever he did worked," Valerie says. Something he wouldn't do was give her a prognosis. "I asked, and he said, 'There's no point in statistics.' So then I asked him, what about this famous five-year thing, what are the chances of this recurring in five years, and he said, '98 percent.'"[5]

He was not programming death by expectation, as is the case with statistical prognostic statements. He wasn't saying you have six months to live on this treatment, as one doctor told a friend of Chris Sinding's, who had inflammatory breast cancer. Such an odd phrase, Chris muses: "I have a certain number of months here in my doctor's bag, and I'm going to give you this many." Chris says with glee, "That was years ago, and she's still with us."[6]

Valerie's doctor was saying, yes, the cancer will come back, but he wasn't saying, it will come back and kill you on a specified schedule.

"Why would I talk about statistics?" he asked her. "The only thing that matters is that you've got stage 4 and there is no stage 5. We're just going to see how long we can make this stage last, and we're not going to worry about the average population."

"It's only in retrospect I realize that [the first oncologist's] attitude would have meant that I would have been dead in six months if I had stayed with him," Valerie says. "Both because of his attitude and because I wouldn't have gotten the right treatment. . . . He was the one who said pretty much, 'Poor lady, let's give her a mastectomy and morphine and send her home'. . . . I knew very early on that I wanted to fight it, I was willing to do anything that would extend my life, but I realize now that an attitude of someone who has just written me off, I don't know if I would have had the personal courage to defy that."

Valerie was lucky to find a good physician who knew how to deliver a tough message without skewering hope. From his experience and training, he could see that the condition might be hopeless, but that she, the individual, didn't have to be. He enabled Valerie, a patient with late stage cancer, to hold two views: to understand that her situation was bleak but that she could hope, not for a different ultimate outcome, but for a different process in eventually arriving. The hope lies in the journey, not the destination. This is an integral part of successful treatment.

The Hope Foundation at the University of Alberta in Edmonton has research indicating that once patients lose hope, they lose the will to fight and stop participating in their treatment, and that a strong basis for maintaining an optimistic outlook is a good and trusting relationship with their doctor. Other evidence goes further, suggesting that the quality of the doctor-patient relationship has far-reaching effects not only on how patients feel but on how they actually fare; that it has an impact on "symptom resolution, function, physiological measures and pain control."[7] All this puts a hefty burden on doctors.

The informal attention paid to emotional and social needs of patients used to fall to GPs, who often knew their patients from birth to death, those doctors many of us remember from our childhood who could cure all ills, not just physical ones. Or at least help us cope. "He functioned not only as a scientist skilled in the diagnosis and treatment of disease, but also as a priest and a friend."[8] The explosion of high-techery and specialization streamlined such "frills" right out of whole levels of medical care, or so it seemed to breast cancer patients whose treatment was conducted in a limbo where hearts and minds and souls had no part, where a surgeon could say with impunity about his patients, "I don't worry about them after surgery, I just leave all that crap to the chaplains."[9] No longer.

Specialists now are expected to provide a whole lot more than physical medicine. We demand more and more of them at a time when they are being stretched thinner and thinner. We want doctors not only to be good at the physical stuff, but at everything else, too; we want them to be completely on top of the latest research; we want them to know for certain the right course for us; and we want them to support us even if we reject their advice. Most of all, we want them to heal us. We want them always to give us good news, and if they can't do that, we want them to give us the bad news as if it's not so bad, in a way that won't make us lose hope, without destroying us. And we want them to do this without lying, something many medical schools are trying to teach them how to do. This is a tall order.

One of the biggest challenges here is the whole information/decision-making issue: in the last decade or so, information overload has threatened to swamp doctor-patient relations. The huge amount of sheer data directly available to patients is, on the one hand, a positive development, and on the other, just plain scary. Some doctors are frustrated by the amount of information and misinformation patients trundle into their offices and the time it takes to sort it out. It is a dilemma because patients are encouraged to take part in decisions on their treatment, and need information to do so. Doctors are encouraged to lay out the options and advise on choices, but if they do so according to different databases, there will be fallout.

"[Breast cancer] is the most widely published cancer in the world right now," says oncologist Shail Verma. "It concerns and confuses me when women complain, 'I don't know what to do about screening, about my treatment,' . . . from the sheer volume of what's out there, my reaction is, 'God, I don't know what planet you've been on.' I clearly understand how confusing the information is. It's not that there's no information, it's just that there is so much. . . . Tomorrow I will see two new women with breast cancer in my clinic to whom I will probably say it is my view that you should receive chemotherapy and here are the reasons, the data are well recorded in these sites . . . and then still spend the next hour justifying the reason for chemotherapy."[10]

The problem is that a patient's "need to know" is often different from what physicians think she needs to know. It's like a railway track that starts from two opposite ends and is supposed to meet in the middle, but misses.

Dr. Verma works in a large teaching hospital in Ottawa, and he is involved with more than just clinical practice: he runs a clinic for high-risk women as well as clinical trials. It is difficult for him to be constantly second-guessed on a subject to which he has devoted his career. He can't be on top of every single development, yet many patients expect him to be. "That's a totally unrealistic expectation," says Scott Findlay. "I feel for oncologists—a single person simply could not have that expertise, all that information; they'd have to spend 24/7 reading the journals, and they've got patients stacked up the yin-yang waiting to see them; they just can't do it—they are madly swimming just to keep their heads above water as it is."[11]

Then there are the many oncologists who are far more distanced from the research, who work in smaller centres, who try to keep up to date with developments through medical publications, conferences and personal observation in their practice. Exactly as many patients do these days. One such doctor says with beguiling modesty, "Gosh, sometimes I get people in here who know more than I know."[12] He also sees many patients who have quite a different attitude, who look to the doctor for information and firm guidance and are bemused by the expectation that they should be taking part in decisions on their treatment. "My suspicions are that . . . most patients don't want to decide for themselves; many have a very traditional point of view and say to the physician, 'You're the expert, you tell me what I should do. That's why I've come to see you.' Hopefully, the physician who meets with you will give the choices and say, 'Here are the downsides and the upsides, and I feel this is best for you.'"

The final stage in the cancer spectrum, the dying, the palliative, is the stage when doctors want to run and patients can't. "As medical practice grows more sophisticated, more people are living longer with the knowledge that they may be dying. . . . Dying requires emotional and physical stamina from the individual and his family. And the difficulty of negotiating all this has an effect on doctors as well as patients," writes Jerome Groopman in *The New Yorker*.[13] Today, a physician frequently must assume the role that once was the exclusive province of religious authorities, "yet the palliative care he offers is primarily meant to ease physical suffering; he is not trained to alleviate emotional pain."[14]

Who would be a doctor these days? Especially who would be an oncologist who must deal with a disease that keeps smashing doctors back against the ropes. The profession has one of the highest burnout rates in medicine. Many oncologists step back from the fight to go into pure research; some leave the ring altogether. Some burn out but continue to practise, even though they may be doing more harm than good, because they have lost their compassion and humanity. The only way they can cope is to depersonalize their profession. Some keep practising because they love their work and deeply care about their patients. These are the successful ones, not because all their patients get better, but because they recognize the importance of the personal side of medicine. Success, for these doctors, is measured by the means, not just the end. These are the doctors you want to find, the ones who recognize that your expectations of them may be too high, may be unreasonable, but they will still strive to fulfill them. They accept that this is their responsibility; it comes with being a doctor, because their obligations to you must match and balance their influence and power over your journey in the kingdom of the sick.

The drama *Handle with Care: Women Living with Metastatic Breast Cancer* has often been presented at oncology Grand Rounds (regular lectures for physicians)—unlikely venues for a play, but this is no ordinary play. It packs an emotional wallop that most playwrights would kill for, making audiences laugh, gasp, cry, debate and think. The amazing thing is that the genesis for this powerful theatre is research—focus group transcripts about the information needs of women with breast cancer.[15]

"To watch the play is to be in the play," writes Arthur Frank, a cancer survivor and author of *At the Will of the Body*. "This research does what many social scientists talk about in principle but few are able to effect in practice: it listens. . . ."[16] It listens and then speaks in voices and action that make others listen. It doesn't just resonate with women who are dealing with breast cancer, although it certainly does that. It is so comforting to see your own experience validated in this play. It doesn't just tell families and friends what women are experiencing. It speaks as well to doctors. And boy, do they listen.

One of the play's first performances was at oncology Grand Rounds at Sunnybrook Hospital in Toronto in November 1998. The final scene is wrenching: the doctor tells his metastatic patient, Patricia, that there is nothing more that can be done for her.

Then each player comes forward one after the other, a linear chorus, each voice chopping hope into bits: "I am hormonal therapy, and I have nothing more to offer here," says the first. "I am radiation, and I have nothing more to offer here." "I am chemotherapy, and I have nothing more to offer here." "I am your friend, and I am so distressed by what is happening to you. I have nothing more to offer here." Then another actor, her eyes focused on the "doctor" says: "I am seven years of training, residency, fellowship, books, research, articles, your white coat, your Medline searches—and I have nothing more to offer here." Then hope asks, "Is there still room for me here?"

The actor playing the patient, Patricia, becomes an interviewer, curious, interested, detached: "Doctor, how do you cope working with very ill patients?"

"I don't know," [the doctor] responds. He turns, faces the audience. "Who says I am coping?"

The auditorium is silent, and then the applause begins, slowly then building to a roar, going on and on. Finally, when it subsides, a voice emerges from the darkened room: "Don't turn up the lights," it says. "The doctors are crying."[17]

At a later performance, an oncologist said, "I could see myself in this drama. I could see myself in the kind moments, and I could see myself in the asinine moments. We've all had lots of both."[18]

Sometimes it's hard for patients to recognize that doctors are people too, with good days and bad days, with lapses of judgment, with surges of brilliance, with moments of compassion and moments of cold exasperation. Some set themselves up as God, some are expected to be God. The bottom line, though, is that they want you to get better just as much as you do. It's just that some are better at supporting hope than others.

"I love these people, you know," one oncologist told me in conversation about his role with patients. He is a caring man, and it shows. His patients see it. He muses, "I think I've done some good. You can't do everything for everyone, but as long as you do more good than bad. . . ."

꩜

Hope, emotional support: these are two of the age-old concepts gathered into a new basket and given the catchy title "psychosocial" in the literature. The first time I heard the term, Anthony Perkins and the Bates Motel leapt to mind. I have since come to realize that the term is a most useful designation in that it encompasses everything to do with an illness other than the physical. And maybe aspects of the physical, too. It is a new term meaning old things—the threads that weave the human condition, the emotional, spiritual, social and psychological imperatives that influence and direct human behaviour. For a while there, these elements went missing in Western medicine. Health was divorced from everything but the physical, a wedge driven between the body and the mind by technology. But, happily, psychosocial is back.

The literature is full of studies assessing the impact of emotional, spiritual and psychological support of one kind or another on cancer patients. They don't all come up with the same findings, naturally. Some find that quality of life is improved but not length of survival; some find both are improved; some find neither are. This is aggregate numbers talking. A clearer message comes from real people: there is no such thing as a purely physical illness. The implications for women living with breast cancer go beyond mammograms and medical examinations.

The mind is at play always. This is a major tenet of Traditional Chinese Medicine, Ayurvedic and other Eastern medicines; it got kicked aside by the heavy boot of science in the Western world, then thoroughly trampled in the rush to worship technology after the Second World War. It has struggled back. And with it, a growing recognition of all the non-physical issues that influence well-being, even recovery. Such as attitude.

The consensus among many women with breast cancer is that it's important for patients to have attitude, and important for doctors not to. When discussions first surfaced about how an individual's attitude influenced the outcome of her disease, there was much skepticism. Scientists scoffed and doctors discounted. Patients grabbed the idea as a life raft in a sea of powerlessness. Here was something they had some control over. How did it work? Who knew.

But it seemed so, so right, somehow. For some, the life raft came with a hole in it. Didn't matter how upbeat an attitude they maintained, their disease was sinking them. Others investigated the new universe of mind-body connection in health—new at least to Western medicine—and were convinced, especially after discovering that such ideas were not airy-fairy New Age but very much Old Age, grounded in the traditions of medicine that had been around a lot longer than ours.

Medical historians date the advent of modern, or Western, medicine around the mid-1800s, when the physical sciences of biology and anatomy were made possible by new tools. In particular, the microscope provided the window through which to study the building blocks of the human body. Giant strides were made in understanding and treating diseases that had ruled for centuries. Viruses and bacteria were fingered as the culprits in infectious diseases; the human body was parsed down through cell, gene, protein to nano-everything; surgical procedures vastly improved; drugs became the answer to every ailment, from hangnails to heart attacks, but nothing in all this progress has brought cancer to its knees. The inability of science-based medicine to move cancer into the curable category once and for all provides fertile ground in which grows a crop of theories and approaches other than strictly medical. None has a provable connection to defeating the disease but, their proponents argue, neither do the physical therapies.

The theory behind chemotherapy sounds logical—powerful drugs go in and lay waste to cancer cells—but since this doesn't work all the time, for everybody, does this mean that chemotherapy is bunk? Same with mind-body medicine. For some, attitude seems to make a difference. For others, it has no impact. But because we don't understand the connection, and because some people with the feistiest of fighting spirits still die of the disease while others who are miserable and defeatist don't, is that a reason to discard the theory holus-bolus?

Dr. Alastair Cunningham, senior scientist and psychiatrist at the Ontario Cancer Institute, thinks not. Dr. Cunningham has seen cancer from both sides—as a doctor and as a patient. He has developed workbooks as well as imagery and meditation tapes that help people tap into the power of the mind. These compelling and useful tools might not quell cancer cells, but they certainly control much of the baggage cancer brings with it—fear, a sense of loss of control, pain. And who knows what impact such "mind games" have on the physical, as well as the mental, aspects of the disease? "My view," Dr. Cunningham says, "is that healing is something that can be learned and it can come a great deal from within, whereas we tend always to look for it from outside. That's our culture."[19]

Stephen Jay Gould weighs in in favour of attitude, too: "Attitude clearly matters in fighting cancer. We don't know why. . . . But match people with the same cancer for age, class, health, socioeconomic status, and, in general, those with positive attitudes, with a strong will and purpose for living, with commitment to struggle, with an active response to aiding their own treatment and not just a passive acceptance of anything doctors say, tend to live longer."[20] Can't say clearer than that. And this is a scientist speaking.

Other researchers, however, not content to accept anecdotal evidence, decided to put attitude to the litmus test—a controlled study, a challenge since attitude is such a nebulous concept, the variables so uncontrollable. How do you set parameters for "positive"? How long must the feeling last, how strong must it be, how does it manifest itself? The whole exercise is so subjective; it defies the strictures of the scientific method. Nevertheless, almost 30 studies have looked at feelings such as hopelessness, denial, fatalism, optimism, acceptance and hope to see if they shorten or extend life. A meta-analysis of their combined results, published in the *British Medical Journal* in 2002, says they don't affect length of survival, but they do have an impact on quality of survival.[21] A positive attitude doesn't help a patient live longer, just better.

A study specific to breast cancer patients found that a support group doesn't extend survival, but "it improves mood and the perception of pain, particularly in women who are initially more distressed."[22]

Everyone has their own coping styles, and maybe for some, pessimism works better than optimism. It certainly did for Ed Watson, a Winnipegger diagnosed with stomach cancer in 1995. He had no urge to "spray sunshine out my ass," he said. "My doctor told me to be positive, I told him to go to hell. If the cancer was going to kill me, smiling wasn't going to make any difference."[23] My guess is that Ed doesn't belong to a support group. But if he did, he'd find that smiling was not a criterion for entry, that pessimism was allowed, and so was despair, and hope and anger and everything else. What matters, in support groups, is not whether you have a positive attitude, a negative attitude or no attitude at all. What matters is that you can talk about it, that you can express any emotion here in this safe place with people who know exactly where you are at, because they are there, too. You share a language, which is cancer, and it eliminates the need to explain, justify, interpret or defend. You move to another level of communication by virtue of your shared experience. It can be fairly heady, it can be tough, funny, abrasive, informative, liberating, cathartic, exasperating, depressing, heartbreaking—rarely boring.

❧

Valerie's support group meets every week in a residential cancer lodge attached to the hospital where most of the members go for treatment. The only criterion for membership is that you have metastic cancer— of any sort. The morning I went, there were perhaps 12 or 14 women attending, and one man. The meeting started at about 10:30. People wandered in, the facilitator made tea, a tin of cookies was passed around and the conversation drifted back and forth between the cancer world and the "real" world. For this group, those two worlds were the same. Cancer was their world, and this was the place, in this group, in this sunny spacious comfortable room, where the cancer world became the ordinary world. "We do have regular lives, too," one member said. Sometimes that is difficult to remember. "Regular" here is discussion of the pros and cons of a walker or wheelchair rather than of a car or washing machine; how to counteract a radiation burn rather than a sunburn; how to squeeze in a wig fitting between chemotherapy sessions rather than a haircut between work and a dinner date.

Most of the members have metastatic breast cancer. They first started meeting five years before; it was to be an eight-week session. *Five years ago.* And 12 of the original group members are still coming to the meetings. This is perhaps the most tangible evidence of progress in breast cancer treatment. Even a decade ago, women rarely survived metastatic breast cancer for more than a year or two. There were no such things as support groups for metastatic patients, at least groups that lasted long.

"Before this support group," Valerie says, "I thought it was normal not to make any long-term plans after metastatic disease. I didn't renew my orchestra subscription series; why should I? I wouldn't be here. Luckily I was able to get [my tickets] back. The first time I made plans longer than a month in advance was for my trip to Italy last fall. I had booked in the spring, saying to myself, if I'm dead, I won't be going, but if I don't book, I won't be going, so what did I have to lose except the money? . . . Since then, I've stopped hesitating about making long-term plans."

One woman had come to her first meeting most reluctantly and after it was over said that she would never go back. "It was so depressing seeing so many people sick, everyone sitting around talking about cancer." But she did come back, perhaps compelled by the desire to be with people in the same situation as her own. Now she never misses a week.

"For one thing," she says with pride, "we often know more than the oncologists do about something." Maybe not about the big things, but the small things, the important details often overlooked in the high-tech hustle of the cancer treatment centres. For instance, portacatheters. The only man in the group had just had a Port-a-Cath surgically implanted in his chest. When he reported that it really hurt, especially when the nurse tugged the tube from it after a chemotherapy infusion, another patient asked him, "Did you get the cream? It numbs the pain." No one told him about the cream. "Ask for it next time. It helps."

More than information is exchanged here: there is laughter, anger, empathy and totally sinful chocolate biscuits. It is also a place where no explanations and no apologies are needed.

"We get solace and privacy here," one woman said. The kind of privacy that means you can talk openly with other people without fear of frightening them, without unleashing waves of pity or misguided advice, and without crashing headlong into a wall of denial.

"I told my sister, 'When I'm gone, you can have this,'" one woman reported, "and she goes, 'No, no, everything is going to be all right.' As if I was never leaving." Her sister, by denying the reality of the disease, was, without realizing it, adding to its burden. In the group everyone knows that the cancer is real, and it's not pink and pretty. No amount of head-burying is going to make it go away. "People around us need to accept the reality of that, because we are struggling with it, too."

"We understand each other's vulnerabilities," one woman said of the group members, "because they're the same as our own. Often friends and families don't and, though they have the best of intentions, hurt. A friend says to me, 'You look so well,' another way of denying the disease, and I want to say 'Oh yah? Well you should have seen me yesterday when I couldn't even get out of the bath by myself.'" The speaker is young, slim, blonde, pretty, and walks haltingly with a cane. Her Port-a-Cath wound shows just above the neck of her blouse. She is not asking her friend for pity but for recognition. And her friend was trying to be supportive, bolstering her with praise. It's so easy to put a foot wrong when you haven't been there. You never know where the land mine is. "A group like this relieves our families of some of the burden."

Valerie says that the strongest members of this group believe that there is no such thing as remission, that in fact once you have the disease, you've got it. "Now that I'm feeling quite well and able to work part time and generally do what I want, I am afraid of forgetting that I am very ill, that it's going to kill me, maybe not for 10 or 15 years—I hope not, I want to keep going as long as I can—but I call that realistic; someone else might call it depressing. All of us have shared this feeling. I can't imagine life without the constant support from this group."

For many, however, the idea of a formal support group is off-putting; they see it as a place where fears are reinforced. One woman had a friend who was dying of colon cancer. "When I asked her if she wanted to come to our group, she said, 'I can't come, I can't come, it's just not me.'" To talk publicly about her disease was to acknowledge its reality in a way she couldn't handle.

Some avoid support groups because of the pain of losing friends made there. "Do I want to get to know these women? Because there'll be 25 of us. Somebody's going to have a recurrence. Somebody's going to die."[24]

Others see support group meetings as exercises in self-indulgent, touchy-feely rubbish that do no practical good; after all, there is only so much navel-gazing you can stomach, right? An hour with this Ottawa group puts the boot to such criticism. Self-indulgence doesn't get a look-in. And navel-gazing? Forget it.

The day I attended the meeting, the conversation turned to problems regarding the amalgamation of cancer care services into one hospital campus. The restructuring of the Ottawa Regional Cancer Centre was not going smoothly, and the group had become an informal advocacy organization: "What [the administrators] have to realize is improving efficiency doesn't necessarily mean improving patient care," one woman explained.

One "improvement" they were really exercised about was the change in location and the method of administering a bone-strengthener drug that most of them were on. Instead of being provided at two hospital sites in the centre, it was now available at only one. The crunch to one location was causing concern: "There was no place to put me. The waiting room was packed," Valerie said. "When I asked how long this situation would last, they said until the Queensway Carleton Hospital opened its cancer services."

When would that be? In five years.

"I told them I'd be dead by then," she recounted, her eyes suddenly wet with tears. "That's the first time I've ever said that. If they had told me that this change was for medical reasons, I'd accept it, but when it's for administration reasons but they don't admit it, I don't. They should tell us the real reason, treat us as intelligent human beings. They shouldn't patronize us.

Another woman took up the story. "We're hooked up to what some nurses actually call a 'baby bottle'—it does look like that, but come on, give me a break, that's just insulting. It might look like a baby bottle, but that is not milk in there, and how many people go around trailing a 'baby bottle' from a vein in their chest? And then we're told to go away and come back in two and a half hours to have it removed. Or we could take it out ourselves. Have you ever tried to get a tube out of a Port? The 'gripper' is called that for good reason. It's very hard to detach anything from it."

She was in full stride now, growing angrier by the minute. "And it's fine to say to someone, 'Go home and come back in a couple of hours.' But what about those patients who live two or three hours' drive away? And many can't afford or are too sick to drive a car, so to tell them to go away or to go home and come back is telling them to do something that's impossible. This is crazy."

The same day of that meeting I interviewed an oncologist from the same hospital. It was like going from one planet to another. There were shared issues but different interpretations, shared events but different experiences of those same events. It was eerie. He described this same change in procedure with some pride, saying that it was more efficient because it made no sense for the provision of such a drug to take up so much time and space when it wasn't even a cancer therapy drug. His description of the process was different as well: he said that women were hooked up to the "baby bottle,"—a term he actually used—went home with it attached and then a home care nurse came and unhooked them. Not one woman in the support group mentioned a home care nurse.

To get their messages to the higher-ups, the group members had invited someone from the hospital administration staff to discuss restructuring issues. He told them that services were overburdened because metastatic patients were living longer than they used to, so required more care. This wasn't the most tactful thing to say to a support group for metastatic patients. "He doesn't work here any more," one woman said with quiet satisfaction.

"People listen to us," another said. "Our opinion matters. They actually ask us for our opinion, and then people actually listen."

I could understand that. There was such a fierce intelligence among this group—a spare, pared down focus on priorities that perhaps comes from the imperative of an incurable disease.

Twenty years ago in Canada, support groups barely existed. The ones that did were started by patients and were not condoned by medical organizations. In fact, they were actively discouraged in some treatment centres, a mystifying stance that becomes clear when you look at it in the context of the times. Historically, the message about cancer put out by such organizations as the Canadian and American Cancer societies bounced between "cancer kills, so please make a donation" and "cancer can be beaten—so please make a donation."

By the 1950s, relentless optimism prevailed, despite the reality that more women were getting the disease, and more women were dying from it. By the 1970s, the Cancer Society volunteers in the Reach to Recovery support program became the Stepford wives of breast cancer—not by their own choice but because the organization insisted that they present an optimistic and upbeat view of the disease. They were women "who had been there," and it was their role to encourage new patients. They were cast as a walking testimonial to medicine's ability to cure the disease—perfectly normal, good as new after surgery and chemotherapy and radiation. Women who didn't wear a prosthesis to hide a mastectomy or a wig to mask chemo-baldness didn't look "normal," so weren't allowed to volunteer in those days. Some critics claim the program falsified the breast cancer experience by "packaging it as a cosmetic mishap, only slightly more serious than a broken fingernail."[25] Another requirement of these volunteers was a positive attitude to conventional therapy. The subliminal message was that such successful interventions took care of everything. So why would anyone need a support group, the very existence of which would suggest there might be physical or psychological repercussions to the disease, that "normal" might go no deeper than a pretty scarf and a fake bustline. We, and the organizations, have come a long way since then.

Now, most cancer treatment centres have support groups running on the premises, and outside the medical setting, across Canada, are hundreds of groups run by survivors and survivor organizations. In Ontario alone, there is a formal network of more than 70 breast cancer support groups.

Dragon boating might be considered a version of a support group. In 1996, a sports medicine research team at the University of British Columbia, led by Dr. Don McKenzie, went nose to nose with the conventional wisdom that after breast cancer surgery and radiation, women should restrict strenuous upper body exercise so as not to develop lymphedema. He recruited, trained and monitored a small group of breast cancer survivors in the ancient—and strenuous to the extreme—sport of dragon-boat paddling. The women ranged in age from 31 to 62. None of the women developed lymphedema; all thrived, physically as well as emotionally. At their first Dragon Boat Festival race, "[they] completed the course with technical skill, energy and emotion—mostly joy. . . . The impact of [dragon boating] on these women has been overwhelming, the physical changes barely keeping pace with the changes in psyche."[26] Now at least 30 communities across Canada boast breast cancer dragon-boat teams.

At the conference in Victoria we were invited to try our hand—and arms and shoulders, in fact, every muscle in our bodies—at dragon boating. It was an amazing experience. We neophytes were interspersed among the experienced paddlers in large magnificent canoes propelled by a crew of from 22 to 26 people, including a steerer and a drummer. A drummer? This was not wallpaper music, this was a deep thrilling throb to set the rhythm for the paddlers. It gets into your soul. We paddled—I use the term loosely—out into the river, and after about a kilometre, we'd stopped whacking into each other and started to pull together. The prow—the dragon's fierce head—lifted out of the water as if alive. We turned to come back upriver and there beside us was another boat, planted, I think, with careful nonchalance by the organizers. The race was on. We would all rather have had heart attacks than stop paddling. We dug deep, lifting and skimming across the water in a harmony that suddenly gripped us all, the beating drum driving us well beyond our individual limits. Forget drugs. This was the supreme high.

Dragon boaters talk of the three Fs the sport brings: friendship, fun and fitness. These translate into support, emotional and physical strength, and a sense of accomplishment—a sense of living joyfully.[27] More than that, it brings with it the rich context of mythology and legend. You are paddling a boat, yes, you are also taming the dragon. Michelle Tocher, author of *How to Ride a Dragon: Women with Breast Cancer Tell Their Stories,* writes about the first time she saw the breast cancer dragon-boat races: "These women were doing more than winning races or even surviving breast cancer. They were surviving despair—celebrating in the face of death, living with the dragon of cancer."[28]

Mary Trafford says that her dragon-boat team "became the support group I never had—we talk about the experience of breast cancer, swap ideas. A couple of women have had reconstructive surgery, and talked about it, and now a couple of other women are considering it . . . and you know, it's just fun, you feel so healthy. . . . It's like being in this very exclusive club. It's like, out of something really bad can come something really good."[29]

When Nicole's cancer came back with such an ugly vengeance, her dragon-boat team prayed for her, laughed with her, meditated for her, raced for her, and won for her. One paddler wrote, "You can bet that for every stroke of the paddle we take, we'll be sending up a little prayer for you."

Another told her, "We're working hard on the dragon boat—maybe I should say dragging boat—sometimes it's slow going! We have several new people to work with. They think 'focus' is a new type of designer eyewear. . . . Anyway, and seriously, we're doing great. Our spirit is strong and our voices loud. I continue to shower you with healing energy and much love." A third sent her greetings, prayers and love from the whole team: ". . . this gift [is] from a dragon-boat team that missed you terribly this year. The Ottawa race was for you, and so, not surprisingly, we came in first. You were in our hearts, minds and spirits."

❧

With support for support groups swelling to such an extent, family and friends may wonder where they fit in. There is a danger here of leaving out the obvious simply because it is so obvious—the support of family and friends is paramount. This is where hope can flourish or wither.

Family and friends have a more difficult role than do doctors because doctors can send you home after an appointment; your husband, your partner, your mother, your friends can't. They must tread softly and be aware of every nuance in mood; they must reassure when they are the most frightened; they must know when to advise or comment and when to shut up; they must ask the tough questions and hear the tougher answers; they must know when to protect and when to back off, when to agree and when to argue; in fact, they must be like Ecclesiastes and know the time for every season. And all the while, struggling with the impotence of not being able to take the disease away from you.

Someone once told me a story I've never forgotten. He was 65 years old, had a five-year-old daughter and had learned just a few weeks before our conversation that he had pancreatic cancer, that his prognosis was bad, that conventional cancer treatment had nothing to offer. He rejected the "bad" part of the message and was searching for something outside the conventional that might stem the tide. He was remarkably cheerful. "I have a story for you," he said. "I was at the hospital two weeks ago and a nurse told me this about a girlfriend who had cancer." His voice dropped to a whisper. "In the breast, I think."

The cancer metastasized to the brain. "She went blind. She became paralyzed on one side, all hunched up." He contorted his body in illustration, his left eye screwed closed, his shoulder lifted and twisted, his hand locked into a claw. I thought then, "Oh rats, he's telling me a joke, a really bad joke. Don't get sucked in. Wait for the punchline." And I prepared my face to smile politely.

He went on. "Her friend, the nurse, said to her, But after all this, you still have your faith?"

"I have, yes. God has been so good to me."

Her friend was astonished. "God has been so good to you? What do you mean? How can you say that? Look at you, you are dying. You're blind. You are paralyzed."

"Yes," the woman answered. "But it could have been my daughter."

No joke. No punchline. Just a father telling a story that illustrated so profoundly his own fear and love for his child. "I would take 50 cancers, as long as it would protect my daughter," he said.

When a parent, a child, a spouse, a partner, a brother, a sister, a friend can't protect someone they love from illness, they take on the dreadful burden of helplessness, having to watch that person suffer, feeling powerless, and inadequate and full of rage and fear.

The support of family and friends, let me say again, is paramount. I have no doubt that I would not be here, 20 years later, if it had not been for my family, for my husband and the kids, my brothers and sisters-in-law, my nieces and nephews, my friends, all who kept picking me up and putting me back together, time and again. They protected me from pain, they made me laugh, they protected me from myself, they gave me my perspective back, which I'd lose regularly, they made me hope, they made life precious.

Valerie Whyte spoke feelingly about how much she relies on her sister's unstinting support; Vladana Sistek talked of her wonderful parents, "who have provided both emotional and financial support, looking after the kids and taking me to appointments and doing housework and all these things I wasn't able to do," and of a friend who was there for her at all the crucial moments: "I have someone in my life now, he lives in his own place, has his own kids, he's been very supportive. He stuck with me through my first bout, then we broke up but remained friends—he wasn't a relationship type of guy—but when the cancer came back, so did he."[30]

Susan Hess describes how her kids carried her through some of the worst moments. "They helped me retain an equilibrium . . . of sorts," she laughs. When her hair started thinning after the first whack of chemotherapy, they helped pull it out because the youngest wanted it for show and tell. When she was completely bald, her oldest son encouraged her to get a tattoo. One day, she was looking at herself in the mirror and commented with bemusement, "I have a really big forehead. I've never noticed that before." One of her kids explained that that was because she had no eyebrows left.

When she was feeling low about her mastectomy, she wasn't allowed much time for self-pity: her youngest child pointed out with the rapier-sharp clarity of youth: "Better to be alive with one breast, than dead with two."

Susan's doctors circled her with love and support. One even sent her his housekeeper for three months. It worked both ways. One told her, "You know, we look forward to your appointments, because you make us feel good."[31]

When Nicole Bruinsma's friends, colleagues and neighbours heard that her cancer had come back, they too circled her with love and support. They scooped her up and her family with a ferocious tender-ness and tenacity, bringing meals, doing the garden, taking the kids. All these people became her extended family. They sent her prayers and healing thoughts; one friend had an entire sweat lodge in Yukon praying for her. "I hope you feel the love," she wrote. One of her patients sent her angels, which she explained were "metaphors (messengers) for the caring, focus, protection, love and support that we direct to those who have meaning and are significant in our lives. . . . I do hope you know that to your patients there is only one person who defines 'Doctor' in its finest tradition: you!"

One friend sent her dried pressed flowers from her garden; another enrolled her in the Sacred Heart Association and sent a certificate listing the spiritual benefits: six daily masses forever celebrated in the Basilica of the Sacred Heart in Rome and the prayers and good works of the Salesians of Don Bosco. All of these acts and prayers and thoughts studded the horror of recurrence with hope and love.

Her own family simply dropped everything to be there for her. Her mother, Antje, put her own life on hold and devoted every hour to her daughter. Her sister, Anda, and brother, Gosse, came from across the world again and again to be with her. One of her nieces sent her the first of a thousand paper cranes: "According to Japanese legend, if you fold a thousand paper cranes, the gods will grant your wish and make you well again. Here's your first one," the note reads, followed by instructions on how to fold a crane. The instructions peter out with a postscript, "Never mind. I'll tell Anneke [Nicole's daughter] how to make them."

Scott's family moved in as backup, weaving another safety net around her and Scott and the girls; Scott's parents, Joan and Chris Findlay, were there for them always. And Scott devoted his life and work to her, switching much of his research to her disease, tirelessly, desperately searching for a treatment that would work . . . at least for a while.

Such emotional support, and the hope that it engenders, is being recognized—again—as a huge component of health and healing; formal support groups, the support of family, friends and doctors are not secondary to treatment; they *are* treatment.

10

OFF THE BEATEN PATH: COMPLEMENTARY AND ALTERNATIVE ROUTES

It has been a most unexpected journey, a most unpredictable journey, a most incredible journey. Without cancer, there is little chance that I would have met you. Without cancer, I'm not sure I truly would have met myself.

—"Writing as a Means of Healing"[1]

W HEN NICOLE was at the first World Conference on Breast Cancer in Kingston, she and Scott met Dr. John Clement, a British-trained physician and medical consultant for the Immuno-Augmentative Therapy (IAT) Clinic, an alternative therapy centre in Freeport, Grand Bahama. We all had dinner together during the conference, along with a teenage brother and sister whose mother was a long-term IAT patient. It was quite a night. The conversation soared into the scientific stratosphere, taken there by probing questions from Nicole and Scott and the energetic and brilliant youngsters devoted to finding a cure for their mother's disease. The daughter had just rollerbladed across Canada to raise money for the cause; her brother had been invited to audit courses in a PhD program even though he was still

210

in high school. They talked that night about their mother's experience at the clinic, and how well she was doing on the IAT regimen, an immunological serum to boost the immune system in order to fight cancer.

After Nicole finished chemotherapy and radiation that year, she went to the Bahamas to check out the clinic. "The sunshine is healing," she wrote at the time. "The sound of the waves is therapeutic. I feel excited about being here. I feel so much hope here. I used to feel if I ever had a recurrence of disease in the form of metastasis that I would take a gun to my head, but now I see there are many alternatives and lots of reasons to have hope."

She interviewed the medical staff, inspected the lab, talked to patients. For future reference, I hope not, she'd said then. Now her cancer was back. Now it was the future.

The sense of hope she'd experienced in the Bahamas three years before was such a contrast to what now was being offered at home. She was in despair. Her choice seemed to be fight or flight. She chose both. She did not give up on the battle; she just concentrated her fight in places where her hope could survive. "I'm not going to take chemo again, what's the use? I'm going to try something else," she told Scott.

In a sense, Nicole was launched into the world of alternative therapies by a conventional oncologist. "Being a physician, she knew what the odds were under conventional therapy," Scott says, "so I'm not 100 percent sure that she would not have gone to IAT anyway, but I know that if [her doctor] had presented the information to her in a different manner, we would have had a much more vigorous debate about her options. We got out of there and she just said, 'I'm going to the Bahamas.'"[2] Because hope thrived there. Some say misplaced or false hope. Others say there is no such thing as false hope.

It was the same appeal that Bill O'Neill, of the Canadian Cancer Research Centre in Ottawa, had for Nicole. Scott remembers a meeting with O'Neill, a man who defies the conventions of the medical establishment with a kind of unholy glee: "What impressed Nicole so much was his supreme confidence. He said, 'You have metastatic disease? Big deal. You know, tell you what. I'll cure your metastatic disease, and you come to work for me,' and I thought, okay, just a second here, where does all this confidence come from? Don't get me wrong. It's not because he's not a scientist or one of the club, I didn't care about that, but just what exactly was the empirical basis of all this confidence?" At that point, Nicole didn't care where it came from. What seemed utter hubris to Scott was manna to Nicole. It gave her hope that metastasis was not the end of the road.

Scott was poleaxed by developments, by the vicious onslaught of her disease and the turn her treatment had taken. When Nicole told him that she wanted to go to the Bahamas instead of embarking on the intensive chemotherapy regimen recommended by her oncologist, he was stunned. "I tried for maybe 20 minutes to talk her out of it: 'Okay, Nicole, I think we should think about this a bit more . . .' but what was I going to do? What was I going to say? I'm a scientist, I don't have much faith in those things, but I couldn't say, 'Nicole, this might be a load of bullshit.' I just couldn't do it. So I said, 'You want to go to the Bahamas? We'll go to the Bahamas. You want to go to Germany? We'll go to Germany. You want to go the moon? We'll go to the moon.'" And that's exactly what they did.

There began a headlong rush, a search that took her across the world in a quest for something that would stem the cancer. Within a week of confirmation of metastatic disease, Nicole's sister Anda flew back home from Hong Kong, although she had just gone there two weeks before to start a new job. Nicole had an oophorectomy, recommended by her oncologist as a way of diminishing hormone stimulation. What her doctor did not recommend was that she travel within days of the operation, especially not to the Bahamas. He wanted her to take hefty and conventional chemotherapy, not some offshore off-the-wall treatment.

She and Scott flew to Freeport four days after her operation. She started the IAT treatment immediately, an intensive course of an immune-booster serum built from the individual patient's blood and healthy blood, the doses adjusted daily depending on the tumour kill rate measured each morning by a blood test. The patient is given a number of ampoules of serum for subcutaneous self-injection each day, ranging from 3 or 4 to 12. It is pretty much a lifetime commitment.

During his time in the Bahamas, Scott studied the clinic records and interviewed staff and other patients, trying to get a handle on just what the serum did. It was hard for him. The treatment had never been subjected to a clinical trial, and the studies that had been done were without firm criteria or established protocols. Anecdotal and empirical evidence existed that many patients had done well for years, but Scott was doubtful of its efficacy with metastatic disease. He offered to help the clinic staff sort and analyze patient data, dating back to 1977 when the clinic opened, but there were too many holes, the information too chaotic to provide the basis for a scientific analysis of success rates. It was a double-edged frustration for him, as a husband and scientist, unable to apply the tools of his training and experience to a treatment that his wife was staking her life on.

Nicole reported almost immediately that she was beginning to feel better, this despite complications to do with her surgery and the fact that she could barely breathe.

When Scott returned to Canada, Nicole's friend Jean arrived in the Bahamas to stay with her. Her leave-taking a week later was a sad one: she told Nicole that she was counting on decades more of friendship. "Remember, we are going to canoe down the Yukon River together at age 70," she said.

Two days later, Nicole's oldest daughter, Anneke, arrived with another friend, Genevieve. I did the cooking, Genevieve said. "We'd buy a big fish, chop it into chunks and throw them into the freezer. Then we'd just eat our way through it, from head to tail." By now, Nicole was proudly reporting that she could swim lengths in the ocean for 26 minutes without stopping. She swam every day. This was a woman whose lungs were so full of cancer they were barely functioning. This was a woman with such determination and will to survive. The reality was that she was getting worse.

Nicole's place in the Bahamas was like a revolving door, friends and family maintaining a lifeline for her. After Anneke and Genevieve returned home, Gosse, Nicole's brother, arrived with Aiden, her middle daughter. The children were her best therapy, but Nicole said that she was of little use to Aiden that week. She had trouble reading her a story at night because she was unable to get to the end of a full sentence without gasping for breath.

It was her youngest daughter, Saraya's, turn to visit next, but it didn't happen because Gosse blew the whistle. Gosse, also a physician, was horrified when he saw Nicole, and phoned Scott immediately: "I don't know what she was like when she came here," he said, "but you've got to get her home, she's going to die down here."

Scott got down there fast. "She came out to meet me at the plane and it was immediately obvious that she'd gone to hell in a handbasket, and I said 'That's it, we're not hanging around here, this is obviously not doing the trick.'" They flew back to Canada immediately; the day after her return, Nicole had a CT scan of the lungs: she was riddled with new cancer.

"Shock and dismay," Nicole described the horror. "The disease had progressed very rapidly in the six weeks. Double the number of nodules. Original ones had doubled in size. Bilateral pleural effusions. And the high resolution film showed lymphangitic carcinomatosis [cancer in the lymphatic organs]. In short, the news could not possibly have been any worse."

One day later, she was on a plane to Germany with her mother, to another alternative therapy institute she'd heard about from a cancer patient in the Bahamas. "It was a very teary goodbye to Scott," she wrote. "I was panicked not to see him for four days. [We were] met by a driver from the institute, who drove us at an average speed of 140 kilometres per hour to Bad Heilbrun, south of Munich, a beautiful setting in the base of the Alps, very '*Sound of Music*-ish.'"

Nicole's sister, Anda, flew to her side again, this time from Hong Kong to Germany. By now Nicole was so ill, she could not lie flat any more, could not breathe, could not eat, was vomiting regularly.

Scott and the girls arrived; friends had worked some kind of miracle and got them airline tickets on points. "It was idyllic, a Bavarian setting, beautiful landscape. . . ." Scott's voice turns hard with sarcasm. "She lasted there less than a week. It was a nightmare. [The institute] had physicians who were incompetent, absolutely hopeless; she continued to deteriorate." It did not have the resources to deal with "medical situations." As if cancer wasn't one.

Nicole was rushed to a small local hospital. "When she arrived," Scott says, "the emergency doctor said, 'Oh Christ, we get all these patients from that place.'" X-rays and an ultrasound determined that Nicole had massive bilateral pleural effusions (fluid in the pleural cavities around the lungs). The doctor stuck a needle into her right side with local anaesthetic only and drained off two litres of fluid in less than two minutes. Nicole commented afterward, "In retrospect, this was very dangerous, as he could [have caused] a massive pulmonary edema (swelling of the lung tissue). I felt the media sternum shift as he did it. The pain was unbelievable." She had so hoped to be relieved of the shortness of breath, but no such luck. Now not only was she still barely able to breathe but she was also in excruciating pain. "That night, I was so hypoxic I was not thinking straight," she recalled. Not enough oxygen was getting to her brain. "Each time I dozed off for even a few minutes, my respirations would slow, hypoxia would start, and I would immediately become restless again and my respirations would quicken again. I am sure that it was the restlessness that kept me alive." Her mother stayed with her all night, as she would do so often in the coming months.

Nicole was so desperately ill by now that the pleural cavity that had been drained the day before was full again, and then it got worse. She had a pericardial effusion—fluid build-up around the heart that could kill her in an instant—and was rushed by ambulance to hospital in

Munich, an hour away. There she was put on a heart monitor in the intensive care unit while the doctors tried to decide what to do.

Nicole had family in the Netherlands, from where her parents had immigrated to Canada in 1954. Her brother, Gosse, worked for a pharmaceutical company in Amsterdam and knew the renowned research oncologist and clinician Dr. H.M. Pinedo, who was on the scientific advisory board for Gosse's company. It was agreed that they had to get Nicole to the Netherlands, to the care of this doctor, and to her family.

But the physicians in Munich said that she couldn't fly anywhere, that she'd die in transit.

After the Bahamas, after Germany, this was the dark side of the moon. "It was the longest night of my life," Nicole wrote later. "I was terrified to be away from Scott even for a few minutes."

A pericardial catheter was inserted to drain the fluid, heavily studded with tumour, from around her heart. She was given Taxotere to try to keep the fluid from building up again, and finally she was deemed stable enough to be airlifted to the Netherlands. On arrival, she was immediately put into an isolation unit. That was when the doctors told Scott to be prepared for the worst—that she likely would not survive the weekend, that he should talk to the girls, tell them. Sudden death was imminent from the huge pressure being exerted on her heart by the build-up of fluid. And the cancer was everywhere. They couldn't give her any more Taxotere right away; they'd just have to watch and wait and see what happened.

⤬

Alternative or complementary breast cancer therapies earn their acceptance in the world of conventional medicine only by going through clinical trials, where scientific evidence separates the wheat from the chaff. If a therapy is not put to such a test, it is condemned to the chaff pile. Anecdotal or empirical evidence is not good enough—

for scientists and conventional doctors, at any rate. It is for patients, though. Conventional medicine is propelled by statistics arrived at through the orderly analysis of controlled studies and clinical trials. Alternative therapies, in the absence of statistics, are propelled by anecdote and hope.

You get breast cancer. It is stage 1, no nodes involved. You have treatment, and the statistics tell you that your prognosis is very good for long-term survival, that 80 percent of women of your age, with your stage and kind of cancer, live to die of something else. Then statistics are palatable; more than that, you hang onto them as assurance that you'll "beat" the disease. Then the cancer comes back, because, if one thing is certain, it's that this disease is unpredictable. By its very nature it erodes the putative certainty offered by statistics. That unpredictability, of course, can be a good thing or a bad thing: good if the disease doesn't come back even though the statistics say it probably will; bad, if you were reassured that it wouldn't and it did. Or you might have started with a stage 3 cancer, whose prognosis, based on statistics, is pretty gloomy. This is when you start rejecting stats; this is when alternative therapies begin to look like the answer: they are often less invasive, and they offer hope for you, the individual, untrammelled by evidence based on the collective.

Here is yet another conundrum: oncologists offer treatments because of the treatments' statistical rating of success; if the treatment doesn't work, the oncologists must urge their patient to abandon faith in those very numbers and perhaps take something far more experimental, that is, something farther back in the clinical trial process, perhaps a phase 2 experiment. The outcome of this therapy could be as questionable as the outcome of an alternative therapy, but because it is under the aegis of a trial, it still falls within the bailiwick of conventional treatment, and therefore is condoned by the establishment. It is at this point that you are encouraged by your doctor to replace your earlier faith in statistics with faith in the system. Some say this is a double standard at work.[3]

Ralph Moss, a tireless crusader in the battle to get alternative therapies a fair hearing, says, "Drugs that are sponsored by big pharmaceutical companies are given first consideration and accelerated approval, then are praised to the skies by an alliance of company publicists, enthusiastic scientists, government officials and compliant media. But when it comes to treatments that originate from individual entrepreneurs or small companies, suspicion reigns. Innovators are often ignored or harassed, and this is especially so if they happen to come from the field of complementary and alternative medicine (CAM)."[4] Big pharmaceutical companies can get approval and market a drug that could be toxic and with no proof that it extends life, while a small entrepreneur often can't afford the prohibitive cost of bringing a drug through the trial system.

※

In the last few years, a sharper distinction has been made between complementary and alternative cancer therapies; complementary therapies being those that patients take along with conventional treatments, alternative therapies being those that patients take instead of conventional treatments. It used to be that pretty much anything outside the realm of surgery, radiation and chemotherapy was considered "alternative" and therefore suspect. This included everything from diet and exercise to psychosocial support, from vitamins to coffee enemas, from acupuncture to colonics, from essiac tea to Traditional Chinese Medicine. Western practitioners protected their training and turf from all comers, new and ancient. But there has been a sea change, slow but gathering momentum, and it's been brought about mostly by patients. Growing independence, better access to information, more information available, willingness to look farther afield, to question therapies that are tough, invasive and uncertain: it is a movement that has created a better informed group able and willing to make choices.

When Vladana Sistek's cancer came back, she struggled with decisions on treatment, and she struggled with a system that seemed to deny her what she felt she needed; she believed that optimum treatment options were being sacrificed to bureaucratic requirements: "They have to follow policy and procedures; they have to give you something before they can give you something else even though they might be aware that it is not as effective. They have to try it and see if you respond to it," she says.[5]

Her solution was to combine conventional treatment with another route: she chose what she felt was the best of both worlds. Six months after the conference where we had first met, Vladana and I had lunch in a coffee shop in the small town of Athens near Brockville, Ontario. I arrived first and watched her making her way slowly from the door through the rowdy lunchtime crowd. She moved with a remarkable serenity, accentuated by the loud voices and crash of dishes being dumped into the clean-up bins. At that point, all I knew was that she had metastatic disease now. Her cancer had come back within a month of her last chemotherapy; it was in her bones; she was dealing with a particularly virulent cancer that had not been slowed down by treatment. And here she came across the room, hesitant but with an aura of peace. Not a demeanour you'd ordinarily associate with advanced cancer.

Vladana recounted what she had been doing in the last two months that had made such a difference: "Right now I feel really good . . . but I don't give all the credit to Xeloda [an oral chemotherapy she was taking] because in my frustration with the medical system . . . I searched the internet and found the Centre for Integrated Healing in Vancouver. I felt that there had to be something more, something as well as, not necessarily instead of."

The Centre for Integrated Healing is a non-profit society that provides a holistic complementary cancer care program. Its philosophy is grounded in the belief that autonomy, personal choice and self-care play an essential role in the healing process.[6]

Vladana and her partner went to Vancouver on a flight arranged by Hope Air, an organization that arranges free flights for patients who need to travel for treatment but can't afford it.[7] They attended the introductory course at the centre, which covered a range of subjects, including information on complementary cancer care, meditation, nutrition, visualization, decision making, vitamins, supplements and meetings with the centre's medical practitioners. Everything the centre offers "is designed to be safely integrated with conventional cancer treatments."[8] "They don't view chemotherapy as something evil," Vladana says.

The centre believes that the process of healing is unique to each individual: what is of great benefit to one person (for example, prayer, meditation, group supportive counselling) may not be of benefit to another. The centre helps patients create their own personalized healing/ recovery plan. Emphasis is placed on decision making; staff at the centre don't tell you what decisions to make, but how to make them.

"They provide tools," Vladana explains. "Some people make decisions based solely on emotion, others on logic, on rational or practical thinking. They don't take into account their gut feelings." At the centre, they encourage integrating all of these approaches, then leaving the issue for a day or two, then coming back to it with a clearer idea of what you really think and feel.

Since she has been at the centre, and incorporated much of what she learned into her approach to recovery, Vladana has noticed a huge reduction in the side effects of her treatment. "[This] comes from a combination of things: the conventional treatment . . . my feelings or state of mind or perspective—and I think the hope is helping."

Laura G. also elected for a combined approach to her treatment. She had a lumpectomy after months of investigation and research and soul searching. During those months, she also did an intense course of acupuncture. Then she was faced with the next decision. The tumour had been very close to the chest wall, and her surgeon was not sure that the margins around it were clear so encouraged her to have more surgery and then radiation. Instead, Laura did more research, and more soul searching. Her instincts, her experience, the information she had gathered, all convinced her this was not the right route for her. She elected, instead, to go to the Immuno-Augmentative Therapy Clinic in the Bahamas, where she took both the immuno-boosting serum and a course of photodynamic therapy (PDT) to replace radiation as a mopping-up exercise. (A less invasive procedure, PDT involves taking a drug called a photosensitizer, which targets cancer cells and makes them sensitive to laser light, eliminating the sensitized cancerous cells. It is a well-established conventional treatment for lung metastasis and is in clinical trials for chest wall breast cancer metastasis.)

The biggest breakthrough in attitudes to complementary therapies—not sudden, not huge, but more like water trickling slowly through a break in the dam—is the growing number of oncologists who are more accepting of their patients' search for things they can do or take that might help, as long as these complementary approaches don't replace, but only accompany, the prescribed methods.

Not all doctors, of course. Some say the right words but are really only paying lip service, because patients are becoming more demanding of open-minded support. Some doctors don't even do that.

Patricia Hurdle tells of an oncologist who helped her decide on her treatment, but not in the way she had expected. "I saw two different oncologists and radiologists for second opinions, and I chose the one I thought I liked the best," Patricia says. "[He was] a youngish man, in his early 40s, straightforward, seemed to listen." It took Patricia months to decide finally not to take chemotherapy after her first diagnosis. The oncologist said, "Well, it's up to you; it's your decision and you've asked so many questions, spent lots of time, so I feel that if that's your choice, then that's your choice."[9]

Patricia decided on a lumpectomy without any adjuvant therapy. Her cancer came back—in the same breast, same spot. "So all the doctors were like, 'See?'" she says. This time she had a mastectomy, then went to see her oncologist again to ask his opinion on chemotherapy at this stage. She was studying in Montana at the time of her recurrence, and the doctors there were pushing hard for her to take it. He wanted her to do the same, but she'd read the literature and it seemed to her that chemo might make a 9 to 10 percent difference to five-year survival, but "given my sister's experience, I wasn't convinced of the benefits, not by a long stretch."

His response? "If you were my wife, I'd hit you." And he walked out of his office.

Since then, Patricia has been going to a naturopath. "She's so empowering—she says, 'We'll work on this together. You know your body better than anyone. I'll bring my expertise and we'll work on this together.' This was what I was hoping would happen with conventional doctors—we'd be partners, and it's only been in the last year [that] I realized they are resources, not partners and never will be, whereas [my naturopath] says, 'Let's go to see different people, see what they diagnose, then we'll pull it all together.'"

Her doctor set up a team and became the coordinator of a network of practitioners. "I needed her support because I felt so let down by regular doctors; you ask a question and it's like you are questioning their whole certification," Patricia says.

One practitioner in the network is a homeopathic doctor. "You walk into her waiting room and it's like night and day compared with the cancer clinic: people are lively and talking and optimistic—they come with incredible diseases, been on . . . horrible drugs, which give them all these other problems. . . . I always leave her place feeling, Oh! Wonderful. Whereas at the cancer clinic, I always have to remember to build a protective bubble, otherwise I leave there a mess, takes me a day to recover."

This is yet another area where you will encounter disagreement. Few question that hope is an essential ingredient to healing; the debate is about its source. Oddly, in some quarters, hope seems to be acceptable only if it rises from within the confines of the conventional world of treatment; if patients seek beyond—and no amount of wagon circling is going to keep them in any more—hope somehow loses its coin and is considered counterfeit.

One oncologist told me what he did when patients tell him they are doing some kind of alternative therapy. "First, I try to inhibit my initial reaction of disdain and curb my hostility and not say, 'This is not how you should be dealing with this,' but basically, it's a fact of life. A significant number of my patients are taking alternative therapies, some of them don't admit to it but . . . do I discard those patients? No. Do I think they are harming themselves doing these therapies? Well, you want to know what they are taking and get information on them, and perhaps see if they have any value."[10]

He uses a checklist when looking at alternative or complementary therapies: a) Does it do harm? b) Is there any proven value to it? c) What is the cost to the patient, both financial and emotional? and d) What is the cost to the patient in terms of lifestyle? "Somebody who has cancer and pursues a cure, he could be bankrupting the family, spending on desperation instead of spending on quality time with family. You want that important closeness. . . . I think that alternative medicine is, in that sense, evil medicine.

"But if you want to compare orthodox medicine with alternative medicine, I'm prepared to say of course we don't have all the answers. When I go in to see a patient I tell them that, but I say if we do this and this and this, it might cure you, it might not, or I may have to tell them that I can't do anything or very little. The natural inclination then is for them to say, well, I'll look for something else. So some do-gooder, or some not so do-gooder who just wants to put money in his pockets, comes along and says, you do this, this and this, and it's very easy and we'll make you all better. That's very attractive to a layperson; you'd jump on it. I might too, who knows. When you are desperate, it's absolutely understandable."

Desperation isn't always part of the equation, although it is a large part for patients whose conventional treatments have failed them. But more and more women are hedging their bets right from the beginning of treatment. Have the surgery, but do acupuncture as well; take the chemotherapy and at the same time drink essiac tea, take mega-vitamin supplements, do relaxation tapes and meditate. In doing this, they are playing a far bigger role in their own treatment. They don't focus just on methods that attack the tumour, directly, physically and hard, a bio-medical model in which "the person or 'self,' play[s] little role in recovery." They are recognizing the benefits of supporting the mind, body and spirit, an emerging "cancer care paradigm, based on a 'person oriented model.'"[11]

Many breast cancer patients figured out the benefits of this approach a long time ago and have had to fight to get recognition that it is more than just a theory to be tolerated, that it is one to be encouraged. And more and more, it is.

Shortly before Susan Hess had a mastectomy, she went outside one night and looked up into the starlit sky. She had an overwhelming feeling that it was going to be okay. She was going to be okay. Where did this feeling come from? She didn't know, but she could not deny its strength and its comfort. About the same time, she was speaking to another friend on the phone, telling her what had been happening to her, and the friend told her, "All the time we've been talking, I've been seeing a vision of a tree with deep, deep roots and healthy green leaves. Like this tree, you have strength; you are going to be well."

Susan says, "I took these two pieces into my heart."[12] They were the best medicine, the best drug, to help her back to health.

Immediately after her diagnosis, she started listening to relaxation tapes—music with a subliminal message. "I listened to them 24 hours a day," she says. "They were my lifeline. I panicked if I had to take off those earphones." In the hospital, when the nurses came to get her for her mastectomy, they told her she had to leave her tapes behind. "No tapes, no surgery," she said. They let her wear her Walkman into the operating room. If you knew Susan, you'd understand their ready capitulation. Susan is small, delicate boned, large eyes in a heart-shaped face. Her soft musical voice, self-deprecating manner, her quirky humour lend an aura of lovely gentleness that is absolutely real. But buried deep is the steel of survival, of independence, an unshakeable faith in the spirit and things spiritual.

A few years ago, even this small shift from the standard approach would not have been brooked. No one would have been allowed into surgery with headphones. Relaxation tapes and meditation exercises were tolerated maybe as harmless, fringe activities, practised by New Age freaks, but certainly not to be encouraged. Now there is growing recognition of the huge impact of such complementary therapies within the mainstream. In fact, it has a name and has spawned a medical discipline: psychosocial oncology. Barry Bultz, an oncologist and director of Psychosocial Resources at the Tom Baker Cancer Centre in Calgary, believes that relieving stress is almost as important as administering drugs to cancer patients. "We need a different paradigm, right from the diagnosis, and not just when a patient is dying," he says.[13] He runs retreat-based programs every two months in Calgary and would like to encourage interest in such programs across the country. It's slow going though, because there is still resistance to the apparent no-brainer that the mind is connected to the body.

Research points to another reason why the health system should welcome such programs: economics. Distress and anxiety in patients actually translate into monetary costs to the system. An Alberta study compared two groups of women with primary breast cancer. One group received normal care; the other took part in a six-week psychosocial treatment program. After two years, it was found that the women in the second group billed 25 percent less than women in the other group. "There's a tremendous body of evidence that there are economic benefits to such interventions," says Dr. Neil Berman, manager of the national cancer co-ordination unit at Health Canada. And enormous benefits to the patient too.[14]

❧

Nicole knew well about the mind-body connection and how it worked in healing. Her friend, Ingrid Meyer, who also has metastatic breast cancer, wrote about Nicole, "'We . . . met frequently in the hospital, where we were both in active treatment. Trained as a physician, Nicole became my teacher, patiently giving me what you might call a 'crash course' in oncology. . . . Repeatedly [though], Nicole stressed that as well as conventional medicine, we had to tap into the power of the mind and spirit."[15]

While Nicole was struggling to hang onto life in Holland, back home, family and friends were frantic with worry and with wanting to be able to do something, anything. One of the things they did was organize a benefit: Christoph Weber, a close friend and colleague of Nicole's, and Jamie Findlay, Scott's brother, spearheaded a group to organize the event to raise money to help Nicole and Scott with the tremendous expenses that were building up. It was at least something tangible they could do. They pulled it together, including a silent auction, in less than a week. The venue was donated—a beautiful ski lodge at Camp Fortune outside Ottawa in the Gatineau Hills, as was the staff for the evening. Several bands gave their time and talent.

People danced, people laughed, people cried. People drank, especially when partway through the evening the venue owners announced that they would donate a dollar to the Nicole Fund from the price of every drink purchased. When we arrived, the parking lot was already half full, more than 400 friends and relations streaming into the lodge. A friend of Nicole's wrote to her about it: "I'm sure [Scott's parents] will tell you all about Saturday night and how you are able to draw a crowd to Camp Fortune even when you are not there!' [It had been here that Nicole had given her first presentation on the need to ban pesticides for cosmetic use, filling the place.] It is so obvious that you have touched and inspired so many people in your life."

Another friend wrote to Nicole just after the event: "'If something comes to life in others because of you, then you have made an approach to immortality.' That's something I found more than 20 years ago, and it has always stayed with me, reminding me of the power each person has in the context of family and community. . . . What I can tell you for certain is that your contribution to the community is immense, in some ways you already know, and certainly other ways you don't."

It was a spontaneous outpouring of love and support and prayers. At the same time, churches in her hometown and elsewhere in Ottawa were holding prayer vigils for her.

Nicole and Scott knew nothing about this event until the morning of it, the Saturday that the doctors expected Nicole not to live through. When they heard, she dictated a message—she was not strong enough to write or even sit up—which was read out by a friend at the event; it was not a letter of farewell, it was a letter of thanks for everyone's help and faith in her recovery. She promised to see everyone soon.

Nicole survived the weekend. She grew stronger. She was able to eat and keep the food down—for the first time in a month. She was allowed to see her children. A few days afterward, she was waiting to be taken back to her room after more tests; she had her medical history file on her lap. "Reading my medical history is a little scary," she wrote. "Metastatic breast cancer to lung and bone, lymphangitic carcino-matosis. Bone metastasis everywhere—sternum, spine, hip. As an MD reading this, I think, wow, this lady is toast. Get out the morphine. As the patient, on the other hand, everything becomes very relative. [I'm] pretty riddled, really. It did throw me for a bit of a loop but undaunted I remain that something will come along that can push those bastards back to whence they came."

While in Holland, Nicole was put under the care of Dr. Pinedo, "the only practising clinical oncologist I've ever met," Scott says, "who had at least a nodding familiarity with every research question/result I ever asked him about, and we discussed dozens." And he would direct Scott to experts, either on his own staff or around the world, who might know more. "It was incredible. I'd go and meet with [him]," Scott says, "and I'd say, 'Have you heard about this research or that research,' and he'd say, Yah, I know a little bit about it, and then he'd pick up the telephone and he'd say, 'Uh, Beppo, I've got someone in my office who wants to talk about aerosol therapy for lung mets, so can you come down?' and in two minutes the lung man would be there with more information. . . . Pinedo is god, and if he said jump, you'd say how high? He could pick up the phone and people would come running. . . ." Pinedo's entire department of clinicians and cancer biologists were integrated to the point where the researchers were often in the clinics.

At the same time that he was doing clinical work (although certainly his patient load is lighter than that of oncologists in Canada), Pinedo was the director of medical oncology, he was attending conferences, consulting with people all over the world, and he still had time for his patients—as people, not numbers. Nicole adored him, respected him. "He knew exactly what to do with her," Scott says. "Maybe his experience is so great, he's seen thousands of patients, he's seen the full range, and he's perceptive enough that after a few minutes he knows this is the hot button and this is the cold button and I'm not going to go there, I'm going to go there. . . ." This doctor, one of the top clinical oncologists in western Europe, had time to talk to Scott about basic research and about every detail of Nicole's treatment. And he had time to talk to Nicole, too, to rebuild her hope.

Soon Nicole was able to go for a short outing in her wheelchair to "see the sun, feel the wind, see the grass and trees and birds," she wrote. Then longer wheelchair walks with Scott's parents, then the big day when she walked with Scott, pushing the wheelchair, not sitting in it. On July 22, just two weeks after the weekend she was supposed to have died, Nicole was discharged from the hospital. She went to stay at a house outside Amsterdam owned by her uncle, a home that quickly filled up with her family, her kids, their cousins, a swirl of life. Now here was a truly idyllic spot.

She wrote about her first night there: "How quickly life moves on. A few days ago I was unable to wrap my head around the next hour of life, [this morning, I was] slowly able to think about tomorrow and now [I'm] already looking a few weeks ahead. Everyone here has been overwhelmingly positive and supportive. . . . Lying in my bed in complete bliss, I finally fell asleep before dinner."

At which there were seven adults and six kids. This was to be the pattern for the rest of the summer; Nicole was surrounded by love and support from those around her, and from those across the globe. She described how she felt, with a kind of awe: "I still rather enjoy one day at a time, with each new joy and success. I cannot begin even to explain the intense joy I get from daily pleasures such as eating, showering or even looking at a flower. . . . I love my life so intensely I am fully enjoying every moment of it that I have. . . . But I am now back in the ring (almost down for the count last week) and I'm ready for a hell of a fight."

After six weeks, tests showed that the cancer growth had been arrested, that tumour activity in her lungs may have even regressed.

After just under two months, Nicole was finally strong enough to return to Canada. "Am deliriously happy about going home," she wrote. Sad to miss Saraya's first day at school by one day, but happy to be back in time for Aiden's and Anneke's. To be back in her own life with Scott and her daughters. That was all that mattered.

"She went from death's door," Scott says. "and by September, she was feeling damn perky and in October, she said to me, 'I feel like I don't have any disease.' She felt like a million bucks."

Later that month, on one of those snappy sunlit afternoons full of light and promise, not only of winter coming but of the natural progression of the seasons, we were at our family cabin in Gatineau Park, cutting and stacking firewood. The leaves were in their final glory, a dance of colour before the sere days of November. It's a haphazard annual affair, this wood-cutting ritual: a potluck picnic, a clean-out of mouse-ridden mattresses, lots of chatter and counter-instructions, a stitch in the weave of traditions, the various tasks moving down through the generations. Scott had run by, on his way to the top of Excelsior, a steep trail that would have most of us on our knees the last few yards. He would be back shortly to join the work and wander brigade.

We'd formed a chain—the choppers, splitting the birch and maple, the carriers, and the stackers, who got to crouch in the low-ceilinged cellar whacking themselves senseless off the floor beams. The cabin sits on the side of a wooded hill overlooking one of the main park trails. We could see flashes of colour down through the trees as hikers passed by, could hear their voices occasionally. I had just finished a stacking stint and had come round the corner of the porch, trying to straighten up without breaking, when I saw one of the flashes of colour turn up our trail, a steepish clamber to the cabin. It was Nicole, bouncing up the hill, indeed looking like a million bucks. She had hiked over from her house in Chelsea, a good three kilometres distant, to join the activities, a life-time away from the bleak days of July. Metastatic can be full of miracles.

Nicole's journey from the day she thought hope had died to this day had taken a tough, circuitous route. Some would say that the swing through alternative therapy territory had been a dangerous and unnecessary detour to get where she was that October. Who's to know? She ended up with a great doctor and a particular treatment regimen in Holland, at the very time she needed him and it most. It was a regimen not available to her in Canada. How did this happen? Happenstance, coincidence? "Serendipity?" Scott asks. "I have no idea. I have no idea. Dr. Pinedo is probably Europe's top oncologist, and [Nicole] would never have gotten to him . . . so in that sense that's the silver lining of going to Germany, and we wouldn't have gone to Germany if we hadn't gone to IAT . . . then we got to Holland and the experience there was just . . . I can't say enough good things about it, it was remarkable, absolutely remarkable. . . ."

But how did Nicole survive the odds that weekend before she even got to Pinedo? Was it the Taxotere? Oncologists would certainly say yes. Was it a miracle wrought by the power of prayer? People with faith would say yes. Was it the power of love? Her friends and family would say oh yes, that must be part of it. Was it her own will to live, to be here a bit longer for Scott and for her children? Wives and mothers would say yes. Or was it the power of hope, arguably the strongest therapy of all? No one can say for certain. Perhaps it was a combination of all these things.

11

JOURNEY'S END: SURVIVING BREAST CANCER

There is a land of the living and a land of the dead and the bridge is love, the only survival, the only meaning.
—Thornton Wilder, *The Bridge of San Luis Rey*[1]

JUST AS THERE ARE 50 ways and more of responding to a diagnosis of breast cancer, there are as many ways of dealing with the journey it embarks you on. When your treatments are finished—you hope for good and forever—you might manage to go back to your old life, shaken but determined to pick up where breast cancer forced you into a detour. Or you might move on to a different kind of life, using your experience as a launch in new directions; you might volunteer to fundraise or help out in a cancer centre or visit patients—volunteering on the small stage. You might venture into the public arena, speaking out for change in the health care system and on social and support issues outside it. You might ratchet up a notch or two and become an activist, wear a button that is not pink and pretty but that says "cancer sucks," and join the many women and men who fight,

232

write, speak, advocate—who have turned their disease into a cause, or even a career.

And if your disease comes back, you might still do all these things for as long as it permits; I am deeply in awe of those women who can maintain such a generosity of spirit, who continue to fight for others while engaged in such a personal battle themselves.

Or you might do none of these things but just keep quietly battling the disease on a private and personal level each time it comes back, and even if it doesn't.

My mother canvassed to raise money for the Canadian Cancer Society, both before and after she had breast cancer. After her mastectomy, after other women had helped her cope, Carole LeBlanc became a Reach to Recovery volunteer. Patricia Hurdle uses music—voice and harp—to help patients contend with fear and pain, especially at the end of life. "When curing is impossible, music can still bring healing in ways that medicine and words cannot."[2] Voice and harp—the music of angels, of medieval monks, of Hamlet's departure from this earth.

Following her diagnosis and treatment, Barb Crooks started a breast cancer support group, then almost six years after her second mastectomy, she had full reconstruction, because no one she knew had had it done in her community and she thought someone should. So other women would know what it entailed. "You know," she says, "after my diagnosis I felt that this was what I was supposed to be doing with my life. I saw my role was to help other women with this horrible disease."[3] She talks about this almost as if it were a calling. Not boastful, just stating a fact.

When Susan Hess was diagnosed, "I screamed and wept and screamed non-stop for two weeks," she says.[4] But Susan doesn't lie down and give up; there is a pattern evident in her life. When confronted by a personal grief or tragedy, she fights to the surface, does what has to be done, and then takes the battle to a higher level. She ends up fighting for equilibrium and solutions not only in her private life—for herself and her family—but in the public arena, for other people struggling with similar afflictions. When it became apparent that one of her daughters was suffering from a mental illness that slowed her cognitive development, Susan threw herself not only into the private struggle to help and protect her daughter through her growing up years and on, she launched a public campaign to increase awareness of children's mental illness and to change the system at the public policy level.

When breast cancer took her down, the same pattern emerged. "I made a conscious choice," she says. "I would not be a victim. I read everything I could find, I did relaxation exercises, I did visualization, anything to help me through it. At first, I did all these things to get myself through chemotherapy, but soon I realized I would always need these techniques."

At the end of her treatment, she refocused, directing her energy outside herself again. And just as she has done in the arena of children's mental health, she moved into the breast cancer community, volunteering her time and determination to help other women struggling with the disease.

Valerie Whyte and her metastatic cancer support group went into battle for all cancer patients in their treatment centre, taking on the administrators and making them listen, fighting against what they believed was a lie when they were told that changes made because of budget constraints were really made for the good of the patients. The changes may have saved money, but they had increased delays and difficulties in treatment, travel time and stress for the patients. The support group members devoted time and energy to this fight; time and energy in scarce supply because of the disease crowding both out of their lives.

Sharon Hampson of Sharon, Lois and Bram went public about her breast cancer in 1993, a courageous act at that time for a woman in public life, especially in the entertainment industry. This probably did more to help a generation of Canadian women than years of admonitions from the medical community to practise breast self-examination. By speaking out about her disease, Sharon helped rout the stigma of breast cancer for many women. "I don't think she fully realizes the impact she has had on a generation of breast cancer survivors whose children adored her," a friend of mine wrote. "It's somewhat fitting that her charming voice soothed and calmed my own two on many a long car journey and her courage and grace did much the same for me on my own journey."[5] Sharon went on to help found Willow Breast Cancer Support Canada in 1994 and continues not only to ride the roller coaster of this disease on a personal level but to lend her name, time and energy to fight it in the public arena.

And Nicole. Nicole used her experience, her training and her waning energy to fight on the bigger stage even as she battled the disease on the private one. When she decided that the link between pesticides and breast cancer was real, she fought at the grassroots level to bring about change at the political one.

However a woman responds, whatever happens, she is known as a survivor.

A lot of us dislike the term "survivor." First, surviving breast cancer is not a one-off thing. You don't walk away from it as you might from a plane crash that leaves you bloodied but a survivor. You keep having to walk away, whether it comes back or not.

You have to survive the fear of the disease as well as the disease itself: fear of treatments; fear of recurrence; fear of pain; fear that you might miss some amazing new therapy because you didn't go for a second, third or fourth opinion; fear that your friends and family will think you a wimp if you keep harping on about it after your treatment is over; fear that the public is going to get sick of hearing about breast cancer before cures are found and turn attention and dollars to a trendier cause.

You have to survive the anger, ranging from the cosmic anger encompassed in the question, Why me? to the very specific rage at enduring months of chemo only to have the cancer come back. There is the broader anger at the system, when you experience delays, errors or inequities in health care; at the media and fundraisers for their portrayals of breast cancer that might seem so far off the mark, so unreflective of the "lived experience" as researchers call the reality. The first time I encountered that term, I misread "lived" for "livid," which is perhaps equally apt. There is the frustration at the turf wars within the breast cancer community and there is apprehension at the growing clout and control of pharmaceutical companies at every level, from grassroots advocacy groups to government drug approval agencies. That's a lot of anger. That's a lot of surviving.

Being called a survivor suggests that you have done something personal and heroic to overcome breast cancer: you are a hero for accepting the diagnosis, enduring the treatments, "beating" the disease. The thing is, you have little choice about the first two—one woman pointed out the distinction between courageous acts, which are chosen, and getting through cancer, which is not.[6] And to claim victory over a disease so utterly capricious seems a particularly dangerous brand of hubris.

At a fundraising event a few years ago, one of the luminaries on stage asked that all the "survivors" in the audience stand up to be honoured and applauded. The person with me knew I had breast cancer, and I wondered, if I didn't get to my feet, would she think I was ashamed at admitting to it publicly, that the stigma of breast cancer was keeping me glued to my seat? But to stand up and be hailed as a survivor? I'd feel a fraud. All I'd done was endure. Nothing brave or valorous about that. And what about all the women who had died of the disease? Did this mean they were cowards? That they hadn't fought hard enough, hadn't eaten the right things, hadn't had the right attitude, weren't heroes?

On top of that was the very real danger—to me—of attracting the attention of the cancer gods by standing up, an action they could interpret as a boast that I had beaten the disease. And they'd nail me again. I ended up sort of half standing, half crouching in indecision and embarrassment.

If, however, you disconnect "surviving" from the concept of achievement, it can become something else entirely, a learned attribute on how to cope. Arthur Frank calls this "survivorship," which he defines as a "form of craft activity, like penmanship, horsemanship, or seamanship . . . an embodied skill at building something or making something work in a precise and exacting way."[7]

So we are all survivors—not a boast, just a statement—whether we fight publicly, fight privately, or don't fight at all. Because, in our own ways, we have all learned how to cope. We have had no other choice. The women in this book represent the spectrum of all women who have had to deal with the disease, the ones who have had breast cancer, maybe years ago, and hope never to have to face it again; the ones who have heard the other shoe drop and deal with the disease daily; and the ones whom breast cancer has killed. They are all survivors.

Some of the women whose stories are told here have died. Is it dishonest or trite to call them survivors still? Does it trivialize the searing pain, the black hole of grief their deaths have caused in the lives of those who knew and loved them? Does it mock the stark reality of their passing and disguise the raging unfairness of the disease? In one sense, yes, of course it does. But there is another way of looking at it. These women are survivors because their spirits transcend death and live on in those who love them. They have left a legacy either in their work, in their relationships, or in their lives. Breast cancer has taken their bodies, but they live on in love and memory.

❧

The telephone call was from Scott. Again, a February afternoon, the dark winter sky heavy with snow and sorrow.

"Nicole isn't doing well. If you want to see her, you'd better come now."

The last few days had been horror after horror for Nicole. Even with almost constant draining, the fluid build-up around her lungs could not be contained; ferocious pain in her side turned out to be, not more cancer as suspected, but a stent that had worked loose inside her kidney. It took three days to discover this. A mistake with the pain medication had nearly sent her over the edge. One arm was swollen badly from the lymphedema, straining the pressure bandage to its limit. Scott, and Nicole's mother, Antje, had been virtually living at the hospital, staying with her and keeping in constant contact with the doctors. Scott continued frantically to try to find another form of therapy to get her on. She'd worked her way through so many.

After several days of this, Scott was persuaded to go home for a few hours' rest. Nicole had stabilized to a point. She knew where she was; she knew Scott; she knew her mother; she knew her daughters. She also knew that she'd reached her limit.

Antje had fetched a yogurt for her; it would be the first food Nicole had had in days that wasn't by intravenous.

"I guess I have to eat this to build my strength back up," she said. She ate a spoonful or two, and then pushed it aside. Nicole had had enough.

The hospital called Scott almost as soon as he'd reached home. Come back, Nicole has taken a turn for the worse. How many turns can there be for the worse?

After Scott phoned us, we were at the hospital within half an hour. When we asked for Nicole's room number at the information desk, the volunteer knew who and where Nicole was; she did not need to consult the Rolodex. Her expression gave away the sad acknowledgment of why we were there. Nicole had worked in this hospital, had done her residency here, had done so many people so many kindnesses here. She had shepherded my father through the labyrinth of emergency procedures years before, when he had been stricken with a mystifying and excruciatingly painful illness, first to get him admitted, then to get him released. And in the last two years, she had been in the cancer ward so often, a patient herself, on the bumpy ride of treatment successes and failures. Half the hospital knew and loved her.

And now, so many were coming to say goodbye.

The first Christmas after her return from Holland, the low-dose regimen which had been working so well had begun to fail; the cancer cells had built up resistance, and her doctors and Scott were casting about for a new approach. At the end of October, she'd been the old Nicole, vibrant, full of energy, slim and laughing. "I was feeling great in October until mid-November," she said. She hiked the Wolf Trail with her friend Jean, who had come to visit. No problem. She was doing her full yoga routine, including a three-minute headstand. A CT scan at the end of September had shown an almost complete resolution of her pleural effusions. In November, she developed a flu-like illness, then a cough—and the pleural effusions were back. Three courses of antibiotics, a pleural tap, a pneumothorax, a chest tube—it was all starting again.

A month later, at a family party in December, Nicole was hardly recognizable: she walked with a shuffle, not enough energy to lift her feet, her body was swollen with steroids, she had lost her lovely hair again, she'd just had a pleural fluid drain that afternoon, and Scott was convinced that she had a collapsed lung. He wanted to take her to Emergency, but she wouldn't go. This might be her last Christmas and she wasn't going to miss anything. She sat quietly on the couch, watching her daughters tear by at top speed with their cousins, a flurry of little girls and piping voices.

She did have a collapsed lung—and dealt with it the next morning. But she did not give up, would not give up. She felt terrible through the Christmas holidays. Her family—her entire family—came for Christmas. That part was great, a tonic, she said, but her physical and mental state were not good. Slowly, though, she started feeling better again. She and Scott had a New Year's Eve party, with everyone skating on the swimming pool rink. The children swooped round with sparklers in the crackling cold night.

That whole winter and spring she struggled back, skiing more and more, doing things with her kids, going to meetings for the Campaign for Pesticide Reduction, but, she wrote, "I just find I would rather stay home and be with my family. Anything that takes me away from that has to be *very* worthwhile."

She told her oncologist, with whom she had made amends: "Get me as good as in October, then I'll switch to Xeloda, then possibly to a Theratope vaccine." Always there was something more to try. By the spring, she was on another therapy, this time low-dose Taxol. Unlike the almost miraculous Taxotere, it didn't work.

"I really thought it would do the same thing," she said. "It hasn't." Her voice was tired, she looked drawn and discouraged; now she was thin, too thin—her body weight was going up and down like a yo-yo. This was the pattern, a capricious up-down, hope–no hope, shuffle-run over the next months.

By fall, she had rebounded again. At the family Christmas party that year, Nicole was back—the old Nicole, the real Nicole, not the one masked and gowned by disease. She organized a family photo shoot, bossing people into place, joking, full of high spirits.

"What's new, Nicole; what have you been up to?" someone asked.

"You mean, besides dying?" she said brightly.

The year before, Death had been sitting on that couch beside her as she struggled to breathe, as she clung to life. This year, Death was banished, nowhere in sight.

But it was just a temporary reprieve, not a commuted sentence. It was exactly as Christina Sinding wrote about her friend dying of breast cancer: "Our laughter and our hope had banished Death, sent her scuttling from the room. Now, she was with us again, sitting on the couch, drinking our wine. And none of us wanted to look at her face."[8]

When Scott called to say it was time to say goodbye, we could not believe it. Not three weeks before, Nicole had been skiing with friends, seven kilometres, and although every step was a battle, she just kept skiing.

She had struggled back from the brink so often that we had come to assume that she would keep on fighting off the disease, keep on overcoming the crises, rallying, storing up more resilience to counter the resistance of the cancer to each therapy. After all, she had lived far past her statistical prognosis. She was hiking, skiing, swimming out along that right tail beyond the median. We had begun to think she was invincible. Her spirit was. Her body wasn't.

Death came back for Nicole two months after Christmas, late that February afternoon in an Ottawa hospital. She died holding a photo of her three girls. She was 42.

EPILOGUE

Nicole made things change in the world, not for her but for the future and in particular for her daughters.[1]

—Annie Sasco, International Agency for Research
on Cancer, World Health Organization

A PRIVATE FUNERAL was held for Nicole in a small stone chapel at Beechwood Cemetery in Ottawa. It was cold and bleak and raw, weather scripted as carefully as in a Brontë novel for a burial. Her sister, her brother, two of her closest friends, her father-in-law, and then Scott spoke. Hearts broke.

It was almost as cold as the December day a few years before, when the funeral service for Nicole's father had taken place in the same chapel. In a note that she had written to me after his death, she touched on the horror of breast cancer. She wrote, "I had not realized the extent of the anguish you have experienced. . . . It will certainly help me to be a more empathetic doctor in the future." This was three years before she was diagnosed with the disease. She had not needed to get the disease herself to be the most empathetic and caring of doctors.

A public memorial service was held two days later in a large hall at Lakeside Gardens in Britannia, but it was not large enough to hold the hundreds of people who came to remember and honour Nicole. It was testament to how many lives she had touched. It was testament to her skill and empathy as a doctor, commitment as a scientist, generosity and love as a friend.

Her daughters' school choir sang; Aiden played the piano; her daughters' music teacher composed and played a piece, "Are You in Heaven," and a friend composed and read a poem entitled "Nicole's Alphabet" that reflected her exuberance, her love of life.

Family, friends and colleagues paid tribute. Dr. Trevor Hancock, chair of the board of the Canadian Association of Physicians for the Environment (CAPE), of which Nicole had been a founding member, vice-president, and honorary president at the time of her death, said: "She was an inspiration, a model of what physicians should be—a committed activist who could look beyond the immediate causes of disease to the wider environmental, social and political context."

Dr. Hancock announced the establishment of the Nicole Bruinsma Award, "in recognition of her achievements, in celebration of her life, in honour of her goals and in commemoration of her passing." It is to be presented annually to a Canadian physician "who has demonstrated their commitment to the ideals and action that she personified."

At the time of the first presentation of the award a year after Nicole's death, Scott wrote:

> *To me, the physician's responsibility is clear: she must use her privileged position in society, her credibility and her medical expertise, to assist in putting in place institutions, laws, regulations and policies designed to minimize environmental degradation and mitigate the health effects of that which cannot be eliminated. In doing so, she must adhere to Cromwell's principle of good governance and give people not what they want to hear, but what is in their best interests to hear. And these conversations must occur both inside and, more importantly, outside her examining room.*
>
> *Although not explicitly stated, these are the principles on which CAPE was founded. They are also—not surprisingly—principles to*

which Nicole cleaved throughout her professional career as a family physician, but especially in the years following her diagnosis of breast cancer.

Two weeks after Nicole died, Scott received a phone call from Peter Cantley, a senior executive of Loblaws grocery store chain. He had read about Nicole's efforts to end the cosmetic use of chemical pesticides in communities. He told Scott that largely because of her work, Loblaws was discontinuing the sale of chemical pesticides in all its garden centres across Canada by the spring of 2003.

Nicole was posthumously awarded the Canadian Geographic Environment Award in the category of environmental health for her work. In accepting the award for her, Scott said, "Were Nicole here tonight, she would, I think, reluctantly agree [with his words of acceptance]. . . . reluctantly because, on principle, she almost never agreed with anything I said. She is not here: our collective loss is great, her family's loss greater still."

ENDNOTES

Chapter 1: The Black Cats of Breast Cancer

1. Conklin, Geoff. "Cancer and the Environment." *Scientific American* 180 January 1949: 323.

2. Nuland, Sherwin B. *How We Die: Reflections of Life's Final Chapter.* New York: Alfred A. Knopf, 1994. 208.

3. Gladwell, Malcolm. *The Tipping Point: How Little Things Can Make a Big Difference.* 2nd ed. Boston, New York, London: Little, Brown and Company, Back Bay Books, 2002. 9.

4. Findlay, Scott. Interview by Penelope Williams, tape recorder. September 2002.

5. Mirick, Dana K., Scott Davis, and David B. Thomas. "Antiperspirant Use and the Risk of Breast Cancer." *Journal of the National Cancer Institute* 94(20) (16 October 2002): 1578–1580.

6. La Vecchia, C., and A. Tavani. "Hair Dyes and Lymphoid Neoplasms: An Update." *European Journal of Cancer Prevention* 11(5) (October 2002): 409–412.

7. American Academy of Dermatology website. <http://www.aad.org>. Accessed 27 August 2002.

8. Nelson, Odile. "Study Links Night Lighting to Risk of Breast Cancer." *National Post* 8 June 2002.

9. Quoted in Davies, Kevin, and Michael White. *Breakthrough: The Race to Find the Breast Cancer Gene.* New York: John Wiley and Sons, 1996. 46.

10. Coalition on Abortion/Breast Cancer. "Abortion Raises Breast Cancer Risk." Pamphlet, n.d.

11. Coalition on Abortion/Breast Cancer website. <http://www.abortionbreast cancer.com/american_cancer_society.htm>. Accessed 23 October 2002.

12. Canadian Cancer website. <www.cancer.ca>, then follow "risk reduction" link. Accessed 24 October 2002.

13. Altman, Roberta, and Michael J. Sarg, M.D. *The Cancer Dictionary.* New York: Facts on File, 1992.

14. Ibid.

15. Quoted in Patterson, James T. *The Dread Disease: Cancer and Modern American Culture.* Cambridge, Mass.: Harvard University Press, 1987. 13.

16. Davies and White. *Breakthrough.* 79.

17. Quoted in Patterson. *The Dread Disease.* 13.

18. Shimkin, Michael. *Contrary to Nature.* Washington, D.C. 1979. Quoted in Patterson. Ibid. 14.

19. Strax, Philip. *Early Detection: Breast Cancer Is Curable.* New York: Harper and Row, 1974. 26.

20. Wynne-Edwards, Katherine. Plenary Session Presentation at Third World Conference on Breast Cancer, Victoria, B.C., 4–8 June 2002.

21. Calle, Eugenia E., Carmen Rodriguez, Kimberly Walker-Thurmond and Michel J. Thun. "Overweight, Obesity, and Mortality from Cancer in a Prospectively Studied Cohort of U.S. Adults." *The New England Journal of Medicine.* 348.17 (24 April 2003): 1625-1638. <http://www.nejm.org>. Accessed 24 April 2003.

22. Brunet, J.S., P. Ghadirian, T.R. Rebbeck, C. Lerman, J.E. Garber, P.N. Tonin, J. Abrahamson, W.D. Foulkes, M. Daly, J. Wagner-Costalas, A. Godwin, O.I. Olopade, R. Moslehi, A. Liede, P.A. Futreal, B.L. Weber, G.M. Lenoir, H.T. Lynch and S.A. Narod. "Effect of Smoking on Breast Cancer in Carriers of Mutant BRCA1 or BRCA2 Genes." *Journal of The National Cancer Institute* 90: 761–766. <http://jncicancerspectrum.oup journals.org>. Accessed 28 July 2003.

23. Couch, Fergus J., James R. Cerhan, Robert A. Vierkant et al. "Cigarette Smoking Increases Risk for Breast Cancer in High-Risk Breast Cancer Families." *Cancer Epidemiology, Biomarkers and Prevention* 10 (April 2001): 327–332. <http://cebp.aacrjournals.org>. Accessed 28 July 2003.

24. Terry, Paul D., Anthony B. Miller and Thomas E. Rohan. "Cigarette Smoking and Breast Cancer Risk: A Long Latency Period?" *International Journal of Cancer* 100 (2002): 723–728.

25. McIlroy, Ann. "Teen Smokers Risk Breast Cancer." *The Globe and Mail* 4 October 2002; Pierre R. Band, Nhu D. Le, Raymond Fang and Michèle Deschamps. "Carcinogenic and Endocrine Disrupting Effects of Cigarette Smoke and Risk of Breast Cancer." *The Lancet* 360 (October 2002): 1044–1049.

26. Davies and White. *Breakthrough.* 43.

27. Profile adapted from Davies and White. 23.

28. Gold, Lois Swirsky, Bruce N. Ames and Thomas H. Slone. "Misconceptions about the Causes of Cancer." In Paustenbach, Dennis J. (ed.), *Human and Ecological Risk Assessment: Theory and Practice.* New York: John Wiley and Sons, 2002. 1415. My emphasis.

29. Varner, Linda. Interview by Penelope Williams, tape recorder. August 2002.

30. Healthnews AP website. <http://wire.ap>. Accessed 17 October 2002; "Cancer Fear Overblown: Study." *The Globe and Mail* 16 October 2002; Metcalfe, Kelly A, and Steven A. Narod. "Breast Cancer Risk Perception Among Women Who Have Undergone Prophylactic Bilateral Mastectomy." *Journal of the National Cancer Institute* 94 (2002): 1564–1569.

31. Verma, Shail. interview by Penelope Williams, tape recorder. March 2003.

32. American Cancer Society website. <www.cancer.org>. Accessed 2 August 2002.

Chapter 2: Searching for the Black Box

1. Findlay, Scott. Interview by Penelope Willliams, tape recorder. December 2002.

2. Breast Cancer Patient. Interview by Penelope Williams, tape recorder. August 2002. Pseudonym used by request.

3. Patterson, James T. *The Dread Disease: Cancer and Modern American Culture.* Cambridge, Mass.: Harvard University Press, 1987. 39.

4. Ibid. 60.

5. Ibid. 60.

6. Huber, Peter W. *Galileo's Revenge: Junk Science in the Courtroom.* New York: Basic Books, 1993. 42.

7. Ibid.

8. Patterson. *The Dread Disease.* 100.

9. "Atomic Bomb Testing Fallout Likely Caused 15,000 Deaths." *USA Today* 28 February 2002. <http://www.rense.com/general20/atom.html>. Accessed 18 October 2002.

10. Breast Cancer Action Montreal website. <www.bcam.qc.ca/news/radiation>. Accessed 22 October 2002.

11. The connection was first made in 1965 by Dr. Ian MacKensie, a Halifax physician, who found that women with tuberculosis who had had numerous chest X-rays had 24 times the breast cancer rate of women not exposed to fluoroscopy.

12. Polyak, Kornelia. "Breast Cancer Gene Discovery." *Exp. Rev. Mol. Med.* (15 August 2002). <http://www.expertreviews.org/0200491Xh.htm>. Accessed 2 September 2002.

13. Davies, Kevin, and Michael White. *Breakthrough: The Race to Find the Breast Cancer Gene.* New York: John Wiley and Sons, 1996. 218.

14. Polyak, "Breast Cancer Gene Discovery." Ibid.

15. Breast Cancer Society of Canada website. <www.bcsc.ca>.

16. Begg, C. "On the Use of Familial Aggregation in Population-Based Case Probands for Calculating Penetrance." *Journal of the National Cancer Institute* 94(16) (21 August 2002): 1221–6. <http://jncicancerspectrum.oup journals.org>. Accessed 28 July 1003.

17. However, this doesn't correct the bias either, though it can still lead to inflated penetrance estimates, according to study author Colin Begg. He argues that all risk factors for breast cancer are over-represented in incident cases of breast cancer. This means that a sample of women who have been diagnosed with breast cancer and who are identified as mutation carriers are more likely to also have other breast cancer risk factors than are similar mutation carriers who are disease-free. (Wang, Linda, and Katherine Arnold. "Risk from Breast Cancer Susceptibility Gene May Be Exaggerated in Most Studies." Press Release. *Journal of the National Cancer Institute* 94(16) (21 August 2002): 1183. <http://jncicancerspectrum.oupjournals.org>. Accessed 28 July 2003.

18. Marcus, Adam. "Breast Cancer Gene Risk May Be Overstated." *Health ScoutNews* 20 August 2002.

19. Findings presented as recently as October 2000 at the annual meeting of the American Society of Human Genetics continued to tout the benefit of both bilateral mastectomies and prophylactic oophorectomies to reduce the risk of breast cancer in women who carry mutations of the BRCA1 or BRCA2 genes. Reuters Health website. <www.reutershealth.com>. Accessed 22 September 2002.

20. Burke, Wylie, and Melissa A. Austin. Editorial: "Genetic Risk in Context: Calculating the Penetrance of BRCA1 and BRCA2 Mutations. *Journal of the National Cancer Institute* 94(16) (21 August 2002): 1185–7. <http://jncicancerspectrum.oupjournals.org>. Accessed 28 July 1003.

21. *ScienceDaily* website. American Association for Cancer Research (13 April 2008) "Identification of BCAR Genes Relevant for Breast Cancer Progression and Endocrine Therapy Resistance." *ScienceDaily*.<http://www. sciencedaily.com/releases/2008/04/. Accessed 14 April 2008.

22. Patterson. *The Dread Disease*. 24.

23. Love, Susan M. *Dr. Susan Love's Breast Book*. 3rd ed. Cambridge, Mass.: Perseus Publishing, 2000. 352.

24. LeBlanc, Carole. Interview by Penelope Williams, tape recorder. August 2002.

25. Marie A., melanoma patient. Interview by Elodie D'Ombrain, tape recorder. Original in French. October 2002.

26. Alexie, Sherman. "What You Pawn, I Will Redeem." *The New Yorker* 21 & 28 April 2003: 169.

27. Peart, Neil. *Ghost Rider: Travels on the Healing Road*. Excerpted in *The*

Ottawa Citizen, section B27, July 2002.

28. Trafford, Mary. Interview by Penelope Williams, tape recorder. December 2002.

29. MacIntosh, Barbara. Interview by Penelope Williams, tape recorder. September 2002.

30. Sistek, Vladana. Interview by Penelope Williams, tape recorder. December 2002.

31. Kim, David. "Breast Cancer: A Comparison between Western Medicine and Traditional Chinese Medicine in the Etiology and Treatment." <www.tdplamp.com/korean/brest.htm>. Accessed 30 April 2003.

32. Hess, Susan. Interview by Penelope Williams, notes. November 2002.

33. Weiss, Rick. "Gene Role Limited as Cancer Cause: Environmental Factors Are More Determinant, Study Finds." *Herald Tribune* (International Edition) 14 July 2000.

34. Ibid.

35. Described by Steingraber, Sandra. *Living Downstream: An Ecologist Looks at Cancer and the Environment.* Reading, Mass.: Addison-Wesley Publishing. 1997. 16.

36. Ibid. 27.

37. Hurdle, Patricia. Interview by Penelope Williams, tape recorder. July 2002.

38. Rogers, Gerry, director. *My Left Breast: An Unusual Film About Breast Cancer.* Pope Productions Ltd. For information: <www.myleftbreast.com>.

39. Rogers, Gerry. Personal conversation with Penelope Williams. World Conference on Breast Cancer, Victoria, B.C., June 2–5, 2002.

40. Mittelsteadt, Martin. "The Killing Fields." *The Globe and Mail* 17 May 2003.

41. When fish with both male and female genitalia started showing up in the Great Lakes system a few years ago, it was suspected that organochlorines were the culprit.

42. Quoted in Mittelstaedt, "The Killing Fields." Ibid.

43. "Global Burden of Cancer." *The Lancet—Oncology Supplement* 2 (1997): 23–26. <http://www.wen.org.uk/health/PBCOM/envfac1.htm>. Accessed 1 June 2003.

44. Reported in Steingraber. *Living Downstream.* 60.

45. The International Agency for Research on Cancer. *Biennial Report 2000–2001.* Lyon, France: The International Agency for Research on Cancer, 2001, 58. <http://www.iarc.fr>. Accessed 31 May 2003.

46. Chrétien, Jean. Press scrum. 5 September 2002.

47. Ford, Anne Rochon. "Toronto Cancer Prevention Coalition Paper on the

Primary Prevention and Early Detection and Screening of Breast, Ovarian and Cervical Cancer." Transcript. August 2002.

48. Verma, Shail. Interview by Penelope Williams, tape recorder. March 2003.

49. Bruinsma, Nicole. Notes for presentation at the Second World Conference on Breast Cancer, Ottawa, June 2000.

Chapter 3: Crossing the Border

1. Peter Carey. *Thirty Days in Sydney: A Wildly Distorted Account*. London, UK: Bloomsbury, 2001. 63.

2. Hampson, Sharon. Interview by Penelope Williams, telephone. August 2003.

3. Ford, Anne Rochon. "Toronto Cancer Prevention Coalition Paper on the Primary Prevention and Early Detection and Screening of Breast, Ovarian and Cervical Cancer." Manuscript. August 2002.

4. Quoted in Ford. Ibid.

5. Plotkin, David. "Good News and Bad News About Breast Cancer." *The Atlantic Monthly* June 1996. 78.

6. Batt, Sharon. *Beyond Early Detection: A New Look at Breast Cancer*. Montreal, Quebec: DES Action Canada, 1996; updated, 2003.8.

7. US National Institute of Health as quoted in Ville Marie Multidisciplinary Breast Center pamphlet. Montreal. n.d.

8. Love, Susan M. *Dr. Susan Love's Breast Book*. 3rd ed. Cambridge, Mass.: Perseus Publishing, 2000. 313.

9. Baxter, Nancy, Canadian Task Force on Preventive Health Care. "Preventive Health Care, 2001 Update: Should Women Be Routinely Taught Breast Self-examination to Screen for Breast Cancer?" *Canadian Medical Association Journal* 164 (13) 26 June 2001: 1837–1846. <http://www.cmaj.ca/cgi/content/abstract/>. Accessed 17 February 2003.

10. Quoted in Paulson, Joanne. "Some breast cancers don't produce a lump." *The Ottawa Citizen* 2 December 2002.

11. Hurdle, Patricia. Interview by Penelope Williams, tape recorder. July 2002.

12. Breast cancer patient. Interview by Penelope Williams, tape recorder. August 2002. Pseudonym used by request.

13. Frank, Marcia. Interview by Penelope Williams. March 1998.

14. Menand, Louis. "What Comes Naturally." *The New Yorker* 25 November 2002.

15. Low, Gloria, Christina Bancej, Ivo Olivotto et al. "An evaluation of organized breast screening in Canada." Presentation. Reasons for Hope, 2001:

New Developments in Breast Cancer Research. Second Scientific Conference. Sponsored by the Canadian Breast Cancer Research Initiative (Quebec City: May 3-5, 2001) *Presentation Abstracts:* 83.

16. Brownlee, Shannon, and Kathy Brewis. "Screen Scandal." *The Sunday Times Magazine* 7 July 2002: 46.

17. Love. *Dr. Susan Love's Breast Book.* 319.

18. Wright, C.J., and C.B. Mueller. "Screening mammography and public health policy: the need for perspective." *The Lancet* 346 (1995): 29–32.

19. Reasons for Hope, 2001: New Developments in Breast Cancer Research. Second Scientific Conference. Sponsored by the Canadian Breast Cancer Research Initiative (Quebec City: May 3–5, 2001) Plenary Session presentation and discussion, 4 May 2001.

20. Quoted in Kirkey, Sharon. "The Mammography Debate." *The Ottawa Citizen* 12 July 1995.

21. Moss, Ralph. "Are Screening Mammograms Advisable?" *The Moss Reports Newsletter* 16 July 2002. On-line subscription, <http://www.cancerdecisions.com>.

22. Gøetzsche, Peter, and Ole Olsen (Nordic Cochrane Collaboration). "Is Screening for Breast Cancer with Mammography Justifiable?" *The Lancet* 355 (8 January 2000). <http://www.thelancet.com>. Accessed 14 January 2003.

23. Duffy, Stephen W., correspondence. <http://www.thelancet.com>. Accessed 14 January 2003.

24. Gøetzsche, Peter, and Ole Olsen (Nordic Cochrane Collaboration). "Cochrane Review on Screening for Breast Cancer with Mammography." *The Lancet* 358 (10 October 2001). <http://www.thelancet.com>. Accessed 14 January 2003.

25. *New York Times* Editorial (27 January 2002) quoted in Moss, Ralph. "Are Screening Mammograms Advisable?" Ibid.

26. Moss, Ralph. "Are Screening Mammograms Advisable?"

27. Ross, Emma. "Breast Screening Saves Lives: Report." *The Ottawa Citizen* 19 March 2002.

28. Love. *Dr. Susan Love's Breast Book.* 320.

29. Ibid. 321.

30. Ibid.

31. Grossman, Joe. "Canadian Study Fuels Mammogram Debate." UPI Science News on-line. <http://www.upi.com>. Accessed 3 September 2002.

32. Batt. *Beyond Early Detection.* 11.

33. Ibid. 17.

34. Brownlee and Brewis. "Screen Scandal": 49.

35. Ibid. 46.

36. Ibid. 49.

37. For example, in October 2002, a private firm called Z-Tech announced a painless, radiation-free electrical device that fits over each breast, delivering a current equivalent to two flashlight batteries. The theory is that electricity moves more easily through malignant breast tissue than healthy tissue. However, the device is at least two years away from regulatory review, provided it passes the clinical trial planned for it.

38. Brownlee and Brewis. "Screen Scandal": 50.

39. Gelmon, Karen A., and Ivo Olivotto. "The mammography screening debate: time to move on." Commentary, *The Lancet* 359 (16 March 2002).

40. Brownlee and Brewis. "Screen Scandal": 46.

41. Love. *Dr. Susan Love's Breast Book*. 145.

42. Carey. *Thirty Days in Sydney*. 63.

Chapter 4: Treatments of Direct Assault

1. Steingraber, Sandra. *Living Downstream: An Ecologist Looks at Cancer and the Environment*. Reading, Mass.: Addison-Wesley Publishing Company, 1997. 31.

2. "Women on Farms Are 9 Times More Likely to Get Breast Cancer." *The Ottawa Citizen* 13 November 2002.

3. Laura G. Personal communication with Penelope Williams. May 2002. Pseudonym used by request.

4. Hurdle, Patricia. Interview by Penelope Williams, tape recorder. July 2002.

5. Love, Susan M. *Dr. Susan Love's Breast Book*. 3rd ed. Cambridge, Mass.: Perseus Publishing, 2000. 336. My emphasis.

6. Steering Committee on Clinical Practice Guidelines for the Care and Treatment of Breast Cancer. *Questions and Answers on Breast Cancer: A Guide for Women and Their Physicians*. Based on Clinical Practice Guidelines for the Care and Treatment of Breast Cancer. Ottawa: Canadian Medical Association, 1998 (updated 2001). 38

7. Love. *Dr. Susan Love's Breast Book*. 375.

8. Roberge, Roger. Interview by Penelope Williams, tape recorder. August 2002.

9. Love. *Dr. Susan Love's Breast Book*. 324.

10. Ibid. 533.

11. Steering Committee on Clinical Practice Guidelines for the Care and Treatment of Breast Cancer. Guideline #8: "Adjuvant Systemic Therapy for Women with Node-Positive Breast Cancer (2001 update)." *Canadian Medical Association Journal* 158 (3 Suppl). (10 February 1998—update 2001). 51.

12. LeBlanc, Carole. Interview by Penelope Williams, tape recorder. August 2002.

13. Plotkin, David. "Good News and Bad News About Breast Cancer." *The Atlantic Monthly* June 1996: 78.

14. Peck, Peggy. "Breast Cancer Location Linked to Survival." UPI Science News website. (27 September 2002). <http://www.nlm.nih.gov/medlineplus/news>. Accessed 1 October 2002.

15. Love. *Dr. Susan Love's Breast Book.* 334.

16. McConnaughey, Janet. "Protein May Predict Spread of Cancer." Associated Press website. <http:wire.ap>. Accessed 14 November 2002.

17. Porter, Roy. *The Greatest Benefit to Mankind: A Medical History of Humanity.* New York: W.W. Norton, 1997. 603.

18. Patterson, James T. *The Dread Disease: Cancer and Modern American Culture.* Cambridge, Mass.: Harvard University Press, 1987. 29.

19. Porter. *The Greatest Benefit to Mankind.*

20. Donn, Jeff. "Mastectomy, Lump Removal Seem Equal." Associated Press website 2002. <http://wire.ap.org>. Accessed 17 October 2002.

21. Steering Committee on Clinical Practice Guidelines for the Care and Treatment of Breast Cancer. *Questions and Answers on Breast Cancer: A Guide for Women and Their Physicians.* Based on Clinical Practice Guidelines for the Care and Treatment of Breast Cancer. Ottawa: Canadian Medical Association, 1998 (updated 2001). 8.

22. According to Cherokee lore, the animals were angry with humans so had a meeting to think up various diseases to inflict on them. The plants, however, took pity and agreed to help humankind cure the diseases the animals and birds thought up. The Cherokees believe that each plant can heal, but first we must find out for ourselves which disease a plant can cure. And that is how medicine came to be.

23. Love. *Dr. Susan Love's Breast Book.* 380.

24. Patterson. *The Dread Disease.* 305.

25. Bahls, Christine and Mignon Fogarty. "Reining in a Killer Disease." *The Scientist* 16[11] (27 May 2002): 16.

26. BTV Communications. *Reasons for Hope: A Breast Cancer Special.* Television documentary. First broadcast, 2001. Broadcast version quoted, 2003.

27. Quoted in Lemonick, Michael D., and Alice Park. "New Hope for Cancer." *Time*. Canadian edition. 28 May 2002.

28. Weinerman, Dr. Brian, B.C. Cancer Agency. Presentation, Third World Conference on Breast Cancer, Victoria, B.C. June 3–5, 2002.

29. Bahls and Fogarty. "Reining in a Killer Disease." 16.

30. Drum, David. *Making the Chemotherapy Decision*. 2nd ed. Los Angeles: RGA Publishing Group (Lowell House), 1998. 1–2, 10.

Chapter 5: Treatments of Indirect Assault

1. BTV Communications. *Reasons for Hope: A Breast Cancer Special*. Television documentary. First broadcast, 2001. Broadcast version quoted: 2003.

2. Hampson, Sharon. Interview by Penelope Williams, telephone. August 2003.

3. Love, Susan M. *Dr. Susan Love's Breast Book*. 3rd ed. Cambridge, Mass.: Perseus Publishing, 2000. 367.

4. Batt, Sharon. *Patient No More: The Politics of Breast Cancer*. Charlottetown, PEI: gynergy books, 1994. 192.

5. Quoted in ibid. 195.

6. Adapted from Webmd website. <http://my.webmd.com/>. Accessed 10 March 2003.

7. Many challenge this number, claiming that the real percentages have been obfuscated by the method of analysis. Laura Shea. Presentation: "Does the Money Speak Too Loudly?" Third World Conference on Breast Cancer, Victoria, B.C. June 4–8, 2002.

8. IBIS Investigators. "First Results from the International Breast Cancer Intervention Study (IBIS-I): A Randomised Prevention Trial." *The Lancet* 360.9336 (14 September 2002).

9. Kinsinger, Linda S., and Russell Harris. "Chemoprevention of Breast Cancer: A Promising Idea with an Uncertain Future." Commentary in *The Lancet* 360 (14 September 2002).

10. Quoted in Williams, Penelope. *Toxic Treatment: Surviving the Cancer Wars*. Toronto: Key Porter Books, 2001. 295.

11. Ford, Anne Rochon. Toronto Cancer Prevention Coalition Paper on the Primary Prevention and Early Detection and Screening of Breast, Ovarian and Cervical Cancer. Manuscript. August 2002. 21, nt. 36.

12. Ibid. 21.

13. BTV Communications. *Reasons for Hope: A Breast Cancer Special*. Television documentary. First broadcast, 2001. Broadcast version quoted: 2003.

14. Levine, Mark, Jean-Marie Moutquin, Ruth Walton and John Feightner. "Chemoprevention of Breast Cancer: A Joint Guideline from the Canadian Task Force on Preventive Health Care and the Canadian Breast Cancer Initiative's Steering Committee on Clinical Practice Guidelines for the Care and Treatment of Breast Cancer. *The Canadian Medical Association Journal.* 164: 1681–1690. <www.cmaj.ca>. Accessed 5 July 2002.

15. Kinsinger and Harris. "Chemoprevention of Breast Cancer."

16. Levine, Mark, Jean-Marie Moutquin, Ruth Walton and John Feightner. "Chemoprevention of Breast Cancer."

17. Ibid.

18. "Task Force Urges Clinicians and Patients to Discuss Pros and Cons of Taking Prescription Medicines to Reduce Breast Cancer Risk." Press release of the Agency for Healthcare Research and Quality, Rockville, MD. 1 July 2002. <http://www.ahrq.gov/news/press/pr2002/brchempr.htm>. Accessed 3 March 2003.

19. Bastian, Lori A. "Women's Interest in Chemoprevention for Breast Cancer." *Arch Intern Med.* 161 (2001): 1639–1644.

20. Love. *Dr. Susan Love's Breast Book.* 390.

21. Filaroski, P. Douglas. "Scientists Design Stealth Molecule." *Jacksonville Times Union* 1 March 2003. <http://www.jacksonville.com>. Accessed 1 March 2003.

22. Strauss, Stephen. "Switching off Gene Kills Cancer, Study Finds." *The Globe and Mail* 5 July 2002.

23. Ibid.

24. Shields, Carol. *Unless.* Toronto: Random House, 2002. 130.

25. BTV Communications. *Reasons for Hope.* Ibid.

26. Ibid.

27. "Customized Cures." *The Globe and Mail* 19 April 2003: F8.

28. Roberge, Roger. Interview by Penelope Williams, tape recorder. August 2002.

29. BTV Communications. *Reasons for Hope.*

30. Sasko, Annie. Presentation at the First Plenary Session, World Conference on Breast Cancer, Victoria, B.C., June 4–8, 2002.

31. Plotkin, David. "Good News and Bad News about Breast Cancer." *The Atlantic Monthly* June 1996: 74.

32. Reasons for Hope, 2001: New Developments in Breast Cancer Research. Second Scientific Conference. Sponsored by the Canadian Breast Cancer Research Initiative. Opening Plenary Session (Quebec City: May 3–5, 2001).

Chapter 6: Pity the Poor Parsnip

1. Humphreys, Helen. *The Lost Garden.* Toronto: HarperFlamingo Canada. 2002.

2. Laura G. Personal communication with Penelope Williams. July 2002. Pseudonym used by request.

3. Findlay, Scott. E-mail correspondence with Penelope Williams. 15 July 2003.

4. Recht, James. "Experimenting in Africa." Letter in *The New Yorker* 10 March 2003.

5. Sutton, Mark, et al. "Is There a Correlation between the Structure of Hair and Breast Cancer or BRCA1/2 Mutations?" *Reasons for Hope,* 2001: New Developments in Breast Cancer Research. Presentations: 140. Second Scientific Conference. Sponsored by the Canadian Breast Cancer Research Initiative (Quebec City: May 3–5, 2001).

6. Lemonick, Michael D., and Andrew Goldstein. "At Your Own Risk." *Time.* Canadian edition. 22 April 2002: 46.

7. Ibid. In a study of cancer patients, at Harvard Medical School, nearly 75 percent of the subjects did not realize that the trial they were in was investigating a treatment that was non-standard.

8. Oncologist. Interview by Penelope Williams, tape recorder. August 2002. Name withheld by request.

9. Health Canada website. "Information: Clinical Trials." <http://hc-sc.gc.ca/english/media/releases/2001/2001_69ebk1.htm>. Accessed 7 May 2003.

10. *The Lancet* Press Release Archives: "New Study Provides Mixed Report Card on Informed Consent to Cancer Clinical Trials." *The Lancet* 21 (November 2001). <http://www.dfci.harvard.edu/abo/news/pressarchive/112601.asp>. Accessed 7 May 2003.

11. Quoted in Lemonick and Goldstein. "At Your Own Risk": 56.

12. Health Canada website. <http://www.hc-sc.gc.ca/english/media/releases/2001/2001_69ebk1.htm>.

13. Davidson, R.A. "Source of Funding and Outcome of Clinical Trials." *Journal of General Internal Medicine* 1 (1986):155–158. Quoted in Bodenheimer, Thomas. "Uneasy Alliance—Clinical Investigators and the Pharmaceutical Industry." *New England Journal of Medicine* 342. 20. (18 May 2000): 1539–1544.

14. Lemonick and Goldstein. "At Your Own Risk": 51.

15. CBC *Marketplace.* "Drug Trials: Who's Watching the Watchers?" Air date: 18 March 2003.

16. Health Canada website <http://www.hc-sc.gc.ca/hpfb-dgpsa/inspectorate/insp_strat_clin_tria_entire_e.html>. Accessed 7 May 2003.

17. "Children's Cancer Trial Went Ahead without Health Canada Approval." CBC website <http://www.cbc.ca/stories/2003/06/12/cancer_trial030611>. Accessed 12 June 2003.

18. CBC *Marketplace*. "Drug Trials: Who's Watching the Watchers?"

19. Lemonick, Michael D., and Alice Park. "New Hope for Cancer." *Time*. Canadian edition. 28 May 2001.

20. Marron, Kevin. "Patient Dearth Dogs Clinical Trials." *The Globe and Mail* 9 September 2002.

21. Verma, Shail. Interview by Penelope Williams, tape recorder. March 2003.

22. Quoted in Moss, Ralph. *The Moss Reports Newsletter* 7 March 2003. On-line subscription. <http://www.cancerdecisions.com>.

23. Ibid.

24. Mathieu, M.P., ed. *Parexel's Pharmaceutical R & D Statistical Sourcebook 1998*. Waltham, Mass.: Parexel International Corporation, 1999.

25. Tufts Centre for the Study of Drug Development, 30 November 2001 <http://csdd.tufts.edu/NewsEvents/RecentNews>. Accessed 22 January 2003.

26. Gawande, Atul. "Desperate Measures." *The New Yorker* 5 May 2003: 75.

27. Ibid. 74.

28. Huber, Peter W. *Galileo's Revenge: Junk Science in the Courtroom*. New York: Basic Books, 1993. 210.

29. Questions adapted from Anne's Cancer website. <http://annescancer.tripod.com/clinical_trials.html>. Accessed 7 May 2003.

Chapter 7: The New Landscape

1. Ivonoffski, Vrenia. *Ladies in Waiting*. Unpublished script for 23 October 2001 performance, Toronto.

2. Canadian Breast Cancer Foundation Community Research Initiative. *Needs and Issues Relevant to Future Breast Cancer Research in Ontario*. Toronto: Ontario Breast Cancer Community Research Initiative, 2002. 7.

3. Ivonoffski, Vrenia. *Ladies in Waiting*.

4. Trafford, Mary. Interview by Penelope Williams, tape recorder. December 2002.

5. Crooks, Barb. Interview by Penelope Williams, notes. February 2003.

6. Humphreys, Helen. *The Lost Garden*. Toronto: HarperFlamingo Canada: 2002. 95.

7. Gray, Ross and Christina Sinding. *Standing Ovation: Performing Social*

Science Research About Cancer. Walnut Creek, CA: Altamira Press, A Division of Rowman & Littlefield Publishers, Inc. 2002. 85.

8. Recognition of this is embedded in the definition regarding women's health adopted at the UN Women's Conference in 1995: "Women's health involves their emotional, social and physical well-being and is determined by the social, political and economic context of their lives, as well as by biology." Fourth Women's Conference at Beijing in September 1995. *Platform for Action.* Ottawa: Status of Women Canada. It is also the cornerstone of innovative research conducted by the Ontario Breast Cancer Community Research Initiative, a partnership of the Toronto Sunnybrook Regional Cancer Centre, The Centre for Research in Women's Health and the Canadian Breast Cancer Foundation (Ontario chapter).

9. Guérette, Lisette. Interview by Penelope Williams, tape recorder. August 2002.

10. BTV Communications. *Reasons for Hope: A Breast Cancer Special.* Television documentary. First broadcast, 2001. Broadcast version quoted, 2003.

11. Madeleine H. Interview by Penelope Williams, tape recorder. August 2002. Pseudonym used by request.

12. "'Nothing Fit Me': The Information and Support Needs of Canadian Young Women with Breast Cancer." National Consultation with Young Women with Breast Cancer, 2002—Final Report Summary by the Ontario Breast Cancer Community Research Initiative, January 2003: 4. Full report available from the Canadian Breast Cancer Network at 1-800-625-8820.

13. Trussler, Terry. *Uncovering the Gaps: An Inquiry of Breast Care in British Columbia.* Vancouver: Canadian Breast Cancer Foundation, B.C./Yukon Chapter, 2002. 11.

14. LeBlanc, Carole. Interview by Penelope Williams, tape recorder. August 2002.

15. Quoted in Ontario Breast Cancer Community Research Initiative. *Update.* OBC-CRI Newsletter Fall 2003: 3.

16. Gray and Sinding. *Standing Ovation.* 79.

17. Interviews for the Lesbians and Breast Cancer Project, OBC-CRI. Researchers: Christina Sinding and Lisa Barnoff. Toronto: Ontario Breast Cancer Community Research Initiative. 2003.

18. Torassa, Ulyssus. "Higher Breast Cancer Risk for Lesbians Not Borne Out, Study Finds." *San Francisco Chronicle* E-6.28 April 2002. <http://www.sfgate.com/cgi-bin>. Accessed 14 May 2003.

19. Interviews for the Lesbians and Breast Cancer Project.

20. Ibid.

21. Batt, Sharon. *Beyond Early Detection: A New Look at Breast Cancer.* Montreal: DES Action Canada. 1996, updated 2003. 27.

22. Ehrenreich, Barbara. "Welcome to Cancerland: A Mammogram Leads to a Cult of Pink Kitsch." *Harper's Magazine,* November 2001: 45.

23. Unfortunately, public awareness of breast cancer has not yet brought some other "female" cancers into the light. There are no spokespeople or lobby organizations yet to help Marie in her struggle. She is speaking out herself. Marie is 55 years old; at age 23 she had a hysterectomy because cancerous cells were discovered in her cervix. She has never had breast cancer, but two of her four sisters have been diagnosed in the last five years, and she herself has had six lumps removed over the years, all nonmalignant. Cancer danced on the fringes of her life for so long, it seemed only a matter of time until it danced centre stage. In December 1998, it did. A routine physical and Pap smear revealed two cauliflower-like lesions on her labia, near the clitoris: melanoma, probably metastatic. She had surgery almost immediately to remove a large section of the labia, and for the next two years, despite new pigmented areas, seemed cancer-free. Then it came back, this time on the clitoris, which was surgically removed. She was told that this form of melanoma was "a ticking time bomb, which in all likelihood will return in one form or another." Marie's willingness to speak about her disease is helping other women by encouraging them to ensure they have thorough and complete gynaecological exams: "Gynaecologists seldom examine the labia and clitoris during a Pap test or gynaecological examination; and my dermatologist told me that most medical personnel are not familiar with the detection of melanoma of the genitalia," Marie says. Nor do we, as women, look "down there" for any anomalies. Marie's message is that they should. Interview by Elodie d'Ombrain, tape recorder. June 2002. Translation from French.

24. Batt, Sharon. Interview by Penelope Williams, tape recorder. June 2002.

25. Landes, Lynn. "Breast Cancer Money-Go-Round: Pharmaceuticals, Pesticides and Radiation Cause Breast Cancer, While Wealthy Non-Profits and Feds Protect Industry." <http://www.ecotalk.org/BreastCancer.htm>. Accessed 25 November 2002.

26. Orenstein, Susan. "The Selling of Breast Cancer: Is Corporate America's Love Affair with a Disease That Kills 40,000 Women a Year Good Marketing—or Bad Medicine?" February 2003. Website: Business 2.0 Media Inc. <http://www.business2.com/articles/mag/>. Accessed 9 June 2003.

27. Ehrenreich, "Welcome to Cancerland": 46.

28. Batt. Interview by Penelope Williams.

29. Ford, Anne Rochon. Interview by Penelope Williams, tape recorder. November 2002.

30. Campagnolo, Iona, 27th lieutenant-governor of British Columbia.

Opening remarks at the World Conference on Breast Cancer in Victoria, B.C., June 4–8, 2002.

31. Ford. Interview by Penelope Williams.

32. Batt, *Beyond Early Detection.*

Chapter 8: The Other Shoe

1. Gould, Stephen Jay. "The Median Isn't the Message." <http://www. cancer-guide.org>. Accessed 22 August 2002.

2. Findlay, Scott. Interview by Penelope Williams, tape recorder. September 2002.

3. Sistek, Vladana. Interview by Penelope Williams, tape recorder. December 2002.

4. Love, Susan. *Susan Love's Breast Book.* 1995 edition: 476, as quoted in Meyer, Musa. *Advanced Breast Cancer: A Guide to Living with Metastatic Disease.* Sebastopol, CA: O'Reilly & Associates, 1998. 27.

5. Whyte, Valerie. Interview by Penelope Williams, tape recorder. March 2003.

6. Meyer, Ingrid. "Nicole Bruinsma: Dragon-Boat Team Mate and Friend." *Breast Cancer Action Newsletter* 4. (2 April 2002).

7. Meyer, Musa. *Advanced Breast Cancer: A Guide to Living with Metastatic Disease.* Sebastopol, CA: O'Reilly & Associates, 1998. 9.

8. Ibid. 34.

9. Menard, Louis. "What Comes Naturally." *The New Yorker* 25 November 2002: 101.

10. Breast cancer patient quoted in Meyer. *Advanced Breast Cancer.* 20. Emphasis in original.

11. Love, Susan, quoted in Meyer. *Advanced Breast Cancer.* 23.

12. Meyer, Musa. Plenary Presentation, Third World Breast Cancer Conference, Victoria, B.C. 4–8 June 2002.

13. Steering Committee on Clinical Practice Guidelines for the Care and Treatment of Breast Cancer. Guideline #9: "Follow-up after Treatment for Breast Cancer." *Canadian Medical Association Journal* 158 (3 Suppl). (10 February 1998). 65.

14. Trussler, Terry. *Uncovering the Gaps: An Inquiry of Breast Care in British Columbia.* Vancouver: Canadian Breast Cancer Foundation, B.C./Yukon Chapter, 2002. 7.

15. Meyer. *Advanced Breast Cancer.* 112.

16. Ibid. 113.

17. Verma, Shail. Interview by Penelope Williams, tape recorder. March 2003.

18. Meyer. *Advanced Breast Cancer*. 209.

19. Ibid. 107.

20. Norton, Larry. "Evolving Concepts in the Systemic Drug Therapy of Breast Cancer." *Seminars in Oncology* 24. No. 4 (Suppl. 10) 1997. Quoted in ibid. 123.

21. National Cancer Institute (US). "'Dose Dense' Chemotherapy Improves Survival in Breast Cancer Patients, Compared to Conventional Chemotherapy." Press release. <http://cancer.gov>. Accessed 13 April 2003.

22. Ibid.

23. Cancer patient quoted in Meyer. *Advanced Breast Cancer*. 203–204.

24. Quoted in Moss, Ralph. "What is 'Dose-Dense' Chemotherapy?" *The Moss Reports Newsletter*. On-line subscription. <www.CancerDecisions.com>. 21 March 2003.

25. Al-Hajj M, et al. "Prospective Identification of Tumorigenic Breast Cancer Cells." *Proceedings of the National Academy of Sciences* 100(7) (1 April 2003): 3983–8: published online before print as <10.1073/pnas.053029 1100>. Accessed 27 August 2003.

26. Quoted in Moss, Ralph. "Scientists Identify Stem Cells As Hidden Cause of Cancer." *The Moss Reports Newsletter* 81. On-line subscription <www.CancerDecisions.com>. 26 April 2003.

27. Study presented to American Society for Bone and Mineral Research. <http://www.nlm.nih.gov/medlineplus/news/fullstory>. Accessed 25 September 2002.

Chapter 9: Beyond Statistics

1. Ronna Jayne. "Hope and Illness" Hope Foundation website. <http://www.ualberta.ca/HOPE/>. Accessed 25 May 2003.

2. Findlay, Scott. Interview by Penelope Williams, tape recorder. September 2002.

3. Gould, Stephen Jay. "The Median Isn't the Message." <http://www.cancerguide.org>. Accessed 22 August 2002.

4. Menard, Louis. "What Comes Naturally." *The New Yorker*. 25 November 2002: 99.

5. Whyte, Valerie. Interview by Penelope Williams, tape recorder. March 2003.

6. Sinding, Christina. Interview by Penelope Williams, tape recorder. June 2002.

7. Gray, Ross E., Vivek Goel, Margaret I. Fitch, Edmee Franssen and Manon

Labrecque. "Supportive Care Provided by Physicians and Nurses to Women with Breast Cancer: Results from a Population-Based Survey." *Support Care Cancer* 10 (2002): 651.

8. Groopman, Jerome. "Dying Words: How Should Doctors Deliver Bad News?" *The New Yorker* 28 October 2002: 64.

9. Gawande, Atul. "Desperate Measures." *The New Yorker* 5 May 2003: 78.

10. Verma, Shail. Interview by Penelope Williams, tape recorder. March 2003.

11. Findlay, Scott. Interview by Penelope Williams, tape recorder. December 2002.

12. Oncologist. Interview by Penelope Williams, tape recorder. August 2002. Name withheld by request.

13. Groopman, "Dying Words": 64.

14. Ibid. 67.

15. The earliest research-based theatre is usually traced to the work of sociologist Erving Goffman who, 40 years ago, "introduced the metaphor of the stage into sociological discourse," and one researcher, Jim Mienczzakowski, in Australia, has been doing research-derived productions for a decade about schizophrenia, substance abuse and sexual assault. (Gray, Ross and Christina Sinding. *Standing Ovation: Performing Social Science Research About Cancer.* Walnut Creek, CA: Altamira Press, A Division of Rowman & Littlefield Publishers, Inc. 2002: 11.)

16. Gray, Ross, and Christina Sinding. *Standing Ovation: Performing Social Science Research About Cancer.* Walnut Creek, CA: Altamira Press, A Division of Rowman & Littlefield Publishers, Inc. 2002: preface by Arthur Frank.

17. Ibid. 91.

18. Ibid. 99.

19. Quoted in Evenson, Brad. "Optimistic Cancer Patients Don't Live Longer, Study Says." *The Ottawa Citizen* 8 November 2002: D19.

20. Gould, Stephen Jay. "The Median Isn't the Message." Ibid.

21. Evenson, "Optimistic Cancer Patients Don't Live Longer."

22. Goodwin, Pamela J., Molyn Leszcz, Marguerite Ennis et al. "The Effect of Group Psychosocial Support on Survival in Metastatic Breast Cancer." *New England Journal of Medicine* 345.24 (13 December 2001): 1719–1726.

23. Evenson, "Optimistic Cancer Patients Don't Live Longer."

24. Trussler, Terry. *Uncovering the Gaps: An Inquiry of Breast Care in British Columbia.* Vancouver: Canadian Breast Cancer Foundation, B.C./Yukon Chapter, 2002. 34.

25. Batt, Sharon. *Patient No More: The Politics of Breast Cancer.* Charlottetown,

PEI: gynergy books, 1994. 232.

26. McKenzie, Donald D. "Abreast in a Boat—a Race against Breast Cancer." *Canadian Medical Association Journal* 159 (1998): 376–378.

27. Mitchell, Terry. Presentation "Psychosocial Impact of Dragon Boating for Women with Breast Cancer." Ontario Breast Cancer Community Research Initiative Advisory Committee meeting. 30 October 2003.

28. Tocher, Michelle. *How to Ride a Dragon: Women with Breast Cancer Tell Their Stories.* Toronto: Key Porter Books, 2002. 22.

29. Trafford, Mary. Interview by Penelope Williams, tape recorder. December 2002.

30. Sistek, Vladana. Interview by Penelope Williams, tape recorder. December 2002.

31. Hess, Susan. Interview by Penelope Williams, notes. November 2002.

Chapter 10: Off the Beaten Path

1. Presentation handout "Writing as a Means of Healing." Second World Conference on Breast Cancer, Ottawa, Ont. June 2000.

2. Findlay, Scott. Interview by Penelope Williams, tape recorder. September 2002.

3. In December 2002 the Food and Drug Administration (FDA) fast-tracked approval of a drug called Gleevac for patients with chronic myeloid leukemia (CML), stating that its purpose in doing so was to make accessible additional therapies that have proven safe and effective through ongoing research and clinical trials. But according to Ralph Moss, Gleevac trials have not yet proven either its safety or efficacy. The FDA approval was based on a clinical trial that measured improvement in "surrogate markers," not direct measures of patient benefit but test results that are supposed to correlate with patient benefit, he says. Patients on Gleevac did have fewer cancer cells after one year than patients on standard treatment, but a decrease in cancer cells does not necessarily mean an increase in survival. An earlier phase 1 trial of Gleevac showed that cancer cells often develop resistance to this drug just as they commonly do in chemotherapy. According to the FDA, CML patients often live up to 10 years with their disease; Gleevac has had only a 14-month follow-up, too short to measure improved survival. And is it safe? Its manufacturer states that "there are no long-term safety data for Gleevac available." Moss, Ralph. "No Glee over Gleevac." *The Moss Reports Newsletter* 31 December 2002. On-line subscription. <www.CancerDecisions.com>.

4. Ibid.

5. Sistek, Vladana. Interview by Penelope Williams, tape recorder. December 2002.

6. Centre for Integrated Healing website. <http://www.healing.bc.ca/about us_overview.shtml>. Accessed 10 May 2003.

7. Founded in 1986, Hope Air <http://www.hopeair.org>, has arranged more than 35,000 free flights since then.

8. Centre for Integrated Healing. Ibid.

9. Hurdle, Patricia. Interview by Penelope Williams, tape recorder. July 2002.

10. Oncologist. Interview by Penelope Williams, tape recorder. August 2002. Name withheld by request.

11. Centre for Integrated Healing website.

12. Hess, Susan. Interview by Penelope Williams, notes. March 2003.

13. Laucius, Joanne. "Reducing Stress Key to Fighting Cancer." *The Ottawa Citizen* 19 May 2003.

14. Ibid.

15. Meyer, Ingrid. "Nicole Bruinsma: Dragon-Boat Team Mate and Friend." *Breast Cancer Action Newsletter* 4. (2 April 2002).

Chapter 11: Journey's End

1. Wilder, Thorton. *The Bridge of San Luis Rey*. Last line.

2. ABC *Nightline* with Ted Koppel. "The Gift: Chalice of Repose Project." Original air date, 25 December 1996.

3. Crooks, Barb. Interview by Penelope Williams, notes. February 2003.

4. Hess, Susan. Interview by Penelope Williams, tape recorder. November 2002.

5. Wright, Sue. E-mail to Penelope Williams. 10 October 2002.

6. Sinding, Christina, and Ross Gray. "Re-Presenting Survivorship: The Interface between Social Representations and Lived Experiences of Life after Breast Cancer." 2002. Manuscript in progress.

7. Frank, Arthur. "Survivorship as Craft and Conviction: Reflections on Research in Progress," 2002. Unpublished. Department of Sociology, University of Calgary.

8. Gray, Ross, and Christina Sinding. *Standing Ovation: Performing Social Science Research About Cancer*. Walnut Creek, CA: Altamira Press, A Division of Rowman & Littlefield Publishers, Inc. 2002. 184.

Epilogue

1. Sasco, Annie. Personal correspondence to Scott Findlay. March 2002.

INDEX

abortions and breast cancer, 12
Action Chelsea for the Respect of the Environment/Action Chelsea pour le respect de l'environnement (ACRE), 42
Advanced Breast Cancer: A Guide to Living with Metastatic Disease, (*see also* Meyer, Musa) 173
advertising, prescription drugs, 104
advocacy, 157–63
Agent Orange, 39
aging
    psychosocial impact on women with breast cancer, 16, 149–50, 153–55
    risk factor for breast cancer, 16, 33
alcohol consumption and breast cancer, 18
alternative and complementary therapies, 210–25
American Cancer Society, 12, 24, 58, 203
American Medical Association, 58
American Society of Human Genetics, 30
Amiel, H.F., 139
anaesthetics, first use, 87
anastrozole, 107
angiogenesis, 108
anti-angiogenesis drugs, 108
anti-nausea medication, 96
Arimidex, 107
Arius, 112
Aromasin, 107
aromatase inhibitors, 106–7, 119
AstraZeneca, 103, 104, 162

At the Will of the Body, 193
Atomic Bomb Study, 30
atrazine, 39
attitude, impact on healing and quality of life, 184, 195–98
awareness and fundraising campaigns, 156, 160–63, 169
axillary dissection. *See* lymph nodes, excision
Ayurvedic medicine, 195

basal cell carcinoma, 93
Batist, Gerald, 98, 109, 114
Batt, Sharon, 101–2, 157, 160
BCS. *See* lumpectomy
Beitel, Laurie, 52
Berman, Neil, 225
Bernstein, Alan, 117
Bertell, Rosalie, 30, 57–58
big business and breast cancer, 160–63
biological therapies, 177
biomarkers, 85–86
biopsies, 69–71, 79
blood tests as diagnostics for breast cancer, 66
bone marrow transplants, 113, 177
bone strengtheners, 180–83
brachytherapy, 93
bras as risk factors for breast cancer, 11
BRCA1 and BRCA2 (*see also* genes, breast cancer)10, 18, 19, 20
    discovery of, 30–33, 114

Morrow, Monica, 88
Mount Sinai Hospital, Toronto, 112, 114
MRI (magnetic resonance imaging), 46–47, 65–66, 89
Mueller, C.B., 57, 58
My Left Breast: An Unusual Film About Breast Cancer, 38
myths about breast cancer, 10–13

Nagasaki, 86
Narod, Steven, 22, 30
National Cancer Institute (US), 60, 76, 155
National Cancer Institute of Canada, 29, 152
National Forum, 1993, 157
National Institutes of Health, 29
National Surgical Adjuvant Breast and Bowel Project (NSABP), 101, 102, 105, 107, 133–34
National Women's Health Network, 101
naturopathy, 222
Neupogen, 167, 178
neutropenia, 178
New York State Institute for the Study of Malignant Disease, 28
Nielson, Eleanor, 151
nocturnal light and breast cancer, 11
Nolvadex (*see also* tamoxifen), 103
Nordic Cochrane Collaboration, 58, 59
Norton, Larry, 95, 179
Nuland, Sherwin, 6

obesity and breast cancer, 17
occupational exposures. *See* environmental factors and breast cancer
October, breast cancer month, 157, 161, 162
older women and breast cancer, 149–50, 153–55
Olsen, Ole, 58
oncogenes, 85–86
oncologists (*see also* doctor-patient relationships)
  attitudes to alternative and complementary therapies, 221, 222, 223
  coping, 192–94
  psychosocial role, 189–90

O'Neill, Bill, 76, 211–12
Ontario Cancer Institute, 109, 197
oophorectomy, prophylactic (*see also* prevention), 22, 23
organ transplants, 136
organochlorines, 39–40
osteogenic sarcoma, 143
osteoporosis and Evista, 126
Ottawa Regional Cancer Centre, 3, 5, 22, 134, 175, 201

pamidronate, 180, 181, 183
Paracelsus, 90
pathology of tumours, 85–86
patient-doctor relationships. *See* doctor-patient relationships
PCBs, 39
PDT (photodynamic therapy), 221
Peart, Neil, 34
Penn, Linda, 109
pesticides
  and AstraZeneca, 162
  and breast cancer, 37–39, 42
  campaign against cosmetic use, 41, 166, 235, 240
  Loblaws' ban, 244
PET scans (positron emission tomography), 67
pharma funding, 160–63
photodynamic therapy (PDT), 221
pickles, 148
Pinedo, H.M., 216, 227–28, 230, 231
placebo, in clinical trials, 128
portacatheters (Port-a-Cath), 199, 200, 202
post-menopausal women, 91, 107
Pott, Percival, 15
poverty, impact on women with breast cancer (*see also* psychosocial factors; social determinants), 149–51
precancers, 53, 63
precautionary principle, 41
premenopausal women, 85, 153–54
prescription drugs. *See* drugs
prevention, 100–1
  and early detection, 49
  definitions, 48–49
  through hormone therapy, 100–5